YOUR
UNCONSCIOUS
IS SHOWING

YOUR UNCONSCIOUS IS SHOWING

Take Control of Your Life
with the 12 Steps
of Consciousness

DR. COURTNEY TRACY

ST. MARTIN'S
ESSENTIALS
NEW YORK

First published in the United States by St. Martin's Essentials, an imprint of St. Martin's Publishing Group

YOUR UNCONSCIOUS IS SHOWING. Copyright © 2025 by The Truth Seekers, LLC. All rights reserved. Printed in the United States of America. For information, address St. Martin's Publishing Group, 120 Broadway, New York, NY 10271.

www.stmartins.com

Interior illustrations by Courtney Tracy

The Library of Congress Cataloging-in-Publication Data is available upon request.

ISBN 978-1-250-32145-9 (hardcover)
ISBN 978-1-250-32146-6 (ebook)

Our books may be purchased in bulk for promotional, educational, or business use. Please contact your local bookseller or the Macmillan Corporate and Premium Sales Department at 1-800-221-7945, extension 5442, or by email at MacmillanSpecialMarkets@macmillan.com.

First Edition: 2025

10 9 8 7 6 5 4 3 2 1

To Bodhi and Gwen, my children, who inspire me every day.
One of you grew up beside me, the other inside me,
as I wrote this book.

Together, with your dad, Max, the absolute love of my life,
you are my reasons to grow a little more conscious
every single day.

Thank you for loving me, human first.
I promise to do the same.

"The words printed here are concepts.
You must go through the experiences."

—SAINT AUGUSTINE

Contents

Gratitude

First and foremost, I want to express my deepest gratitude to my husband, whose unwavering support and love have been my anchor and sanctuary. As this book comes out, we celebrate twenty years wrapped up in each other.

Without "you," Max, I simply could not be "me." I love you.

To my parents, Ken and Deneen, thank you for life. Through it all, you let me be me. You stayed yourselves, and we're pretty loving, cool people. I'll always be your little girl. I love you both more than you will know.

Tricia and Jeff, thank you for your support and love, and for laying the foundation upon which I build my dreams. (And thanks for the husband. He's so great.)

A special thank you to Sammi Cools, you shaped my Truth Doctor journey in ways only your heart and mind could. You deserve all the things. Keep feeling, it's your strength.

To Jessica Flores, thank you for answering my call that day, and every day. I hope to do the same for all our years. You're the best friend I've ever had, and I'm so proud of you.

CeCe Lyra, my brilliant literary agent, you took a chance on me and embraced my project with a passion and commitment that went beyond my wildest dreams. Your guidance has been instrumental in shaping this book. Thank you for trusting I could make my vision a reality.

To Ceri and Sarah, thank you for being there through the proposal and beginning writing stages, helping me navigate its (and my) complexities with grace and patience.

To Eileen Rothschild and the entire team at St. Martin's, thank you for seeing my vision and trusting me to deliver the full meal you hoped it would be. Your faith in this project has been a source of great motivation and pride.

And to all of the people around the world who see me in my truest form, your acceptance and support embolden me to be my most authentic self. Thank you, humans. I'm so, *so* glad that you exist.

Recover from Being Human

"I can't change."

"I'll never be able to control myself."

"I'm the only one who's like this."

"Being a human is so hard."

You're right. Being a human is hard. (But you're wrong about the rest.)

There are two truths I've learned about the human condition that led to me writing this book. I didn't learn them while getting my master's or doctorate degree to become a therapist. They stem from my own life experiences and from years and years of sitting with other humans, listening to their stories.

They are:

1. Many of us treat ourselves (and/or other people) horribly; and this is because
2. The majority of us are in the dark when it comes to knowing how we function as humans. When we don't understand ourselves, we fundamentally cannot understand others.

It's time to recover from being human.

Recovering from being human isn't about learning how not to be one;

it's about mastering the art of being a better version of yourself, of becoming the best human you can. It's about acknowledging that, although most pop psych articles would tell you differently, you don't need to have experienced profound trauma to find yourself operating on autopilot, with unseen forces controlling your emotions and behaviors. It's simply part of the human condition. Recovering from being human is hearing, maybe for the first time, that being human, in its current state, is a chaotic mess, and often is.

Let's face it: Being human is complex. It involves navigating a world where the stories you tell yourself, the ones often scripted by others or by society at large, shape your identity. It's living with a brain that, with its automatic thoughts and judgments, makes decisions on your behalf without you knowing it. And it's living a life that involves frequently ignoring your body's signals, whether as stress manifesting as physical pain or the gut feelings you dismiss in favor of "logic." Like choosing your partner based on their salary and not how well they treat you.

From the moment you were born, society, along with your family, friends, and the cultural norms you grew up with, started shaping you (even the languages you're taught determine which concepts you learn about—some feelings can only be expressed with a specific word from a specific language). The world and its people have presented you with what they believe you should be like—the roles you should play, the behaviors you should exhibit, and the expectations you should meet. But when it comes to the real, raw essence of human nature, there's a noticeable silence. For most of us, we never had someone sit us down to talk about what's going on inside us—the whirlwind of sensations, thoughts, feelings, and behaviors that make up our inner and outer experiences. And without much help, we've been left to figure out life on our own.

The recovery process from being a human who was never really taught how to "human" involves challenging the narratives handed down to you and asking yourself whether they actually resonate with your deepest of truths and your most important values. It's taking a hard look at the choices and decisions you make daily: Are they truly yours, or are they patterns based on your past, inflicting familiar pain from prior experiences in the here and now? And it's tuning in to your body's wisdom, recognizing that physical sensations and emotions are not just background noise but vital signals guiding you toward your health and well-being.

Who Is Courtney Tracy?

I am a woman who was born in Southern California to two teenagers who fell in love.

My parents fought, never married, and, almost immediately, I lived with a single mother on welfare and food stamps, working multiple jobs. Under her Hispanic military parents' roof, she was trying to raise my younger half brother and me—an emotionally intense, oddly rigid, and deeply thoughtful little girl—as best she could.

When I was seven years old, I scored in the ninety-ninth percentile on the GATE test—the test where kids are deemed "gifted" and "talented" in the education system—but stubbornly refused to continue the program because the classroom was too bright and the teacher was too loud. I also peed myself in class (more than once) because I didn't know how to listen to my body's cues. I never wanted to go back there again.

When I was eight years old, I read my grandfather's copy of *War and Peace*—a 1,300-page philosophical narrative about fate and free will in wartime Russia—from front to back every day throughout the summer and refused to do literally anything else.

When I was ten years old, I went to Disneyland ("the happiest place on Earth") and am sure I had the worst time possible. I had never been to a more overstimulating place in my life.

By thirteen, I had lost my virginity and found out that substances could easily alter how you feel, think, and act. I liked this.

And by fifteen, the year the boy I would end up calling my husband entered my life, I would enter rehab for the first time, unable to control the ways my body, brain, and mind wanted to cope. Rehab worked, and it didn't.

Seven years later, after we had eloped and I was still completely out of control, he gave me an ultimatum (one I write about in this book), and it changed the trajectory of my life forever. It was this year, at twenty-two years old, I finally decided to take control of my life, and, in turn, started my path toward becoming a therapist.

Twelve years, five businesses, four degrees, two kids, and a long-lasting successful marriage later, it's safe to say I've learned how to control myself and my life in ways I never thought possible. I'm not perfect, but as you'll soon come to learn, that's not the point of getting better.

Hi, I'm Dr. Courtney Tracy, a University of Southern California–trained licensed clinical social worker and doctor of clinical psychology in California. I own multiple mental health companies, serve on several nonprofit boards, and am an award-winning content creator known online to an audience of over two million people as "The Truth Doctor." I share my truth to help you share yours, and it's changed the lives of many, many people.

I became a therapist (someone who guides others through mental challenges) because, growing up, I needed nothing more than to understand what was going on inside me, *and* what I could do to help myself that wouldn't cause me or other people pain. I needed education and actionable experiences—the two tools I've given you in this book.

I'm a therapist because we live in a world where people need therapists—a world that moves faster than our bodies can handle, with more fear than our brains can process, and more limitations than opportunities to make our dreams come true.

I'm Dr. Courtney, and I'm a therapist because being a human is hard, I get it, and you shouldn't have to do it alone.

What's Inside This Book?

In this book, I present you with a two-part journey.

In Part I, I will shift your understanding of what it means to be human—with detailed, research-backed evidence that you're far more out of control than you think you are. But don't worry, in Part II, I offer you my 12 Steps of Consciousness—your pathway toward improving the amount of control you have over yourself and your choices. Part I reads like a psychology textbook your best friend (who's also a therapist) wrote, and Part II serves as a guide for changing your life—helping you to notice both bad habits and ones you're not aware of, work toward a plan to change, fix past errors, and then share your truth with others to help them find their own, just like me. I put everything I know into this book, everything that's ever helped my clients, and me.

If you've studied psychology, some ideas in this book will be familiar, while others might be new or explained in a way that helps you really get them. I draw on additional fields of study as well, including physiology, neuroscience, and philosophy (fear not, it's made to be a simple, fun, and worthwhile read). My hope is that my style and the way I present this information to you, combined with the personal parts of my life that I share, can be my contributions, along with the clinicians and researchers who originally developed the theories and concepts presented.

Throughout the 12 Steps, you'll answer questions, complete exercises, and finally experience what it's like to *really* feel alive, know yourself, and make your own choices. Most of the experiential exercises are rooted in science and therapy models shown to reduce many common problems we face as human beings (anxiety, depression, stress, impulsivity, disconnection, trauma responses). For those interested, you can find the links between the experiences and the research-backed modalities in the Appendix.

I believe this book is one of the first to touch *all* the hidden processes inside you—from how your body works to the automatic decisions you make without thinking to the ways your life experiences and life stories alter your behaviors. While the information itself may not be "new," I believe my conceptualization of it is, and I'm confident it will help you.

As you read these pages, you will learn about me as I help you learn about yourself. An exchange of truths where my story, I hope, encourages you to tell someone yours, to teach them the steps I'll soon teach you, to spread truth. Why? Well, Dan Brown said it best in his book *The Lost Symbol*:

> *"The truth has power. And when we hear the truth, even if we don't understand it, we feel that truth resonate within us . . . vibrating with our unconscious wisdom. Perhaps the truth is not learned by us, but rather, the truth is re-called . . . re-membered . . . re-cognized . . . as that which is already inside us."*

PART I:
YOUR UNCONSCIOUS IS SHOWING

1

The New Three-Part Unconscious

Before I became a therapist, I was a bitch.

I'm not saying some therapists can't be bitches because . . . they can. But if you ask me what I do today, I say, "I'm a therapist." Had you asked me fifteen years ago, I would have said, "I'm a bitch." Does that answer make sense? No. But most of what we think, feel, say, and do when we're unhealed, unaware of how we function, and unconsciously defending ourselves against future hurt doesn't make sense. At least not when it comes to how we'd truly like to live our lives.

Bitches *act* like they're in control. Therapists know they're not.[1]

Growing up, I wanted nothing more than to be in control. For over a decade, however, I was the poster child for what you'd label as "out of control." Call her for a good time, they said—not the kind of good time you go to a therapist for, the kind of good time that takes place in a bed. Text her if you're using drugs—not for help getting off them, but for help finding them. I didn't care about people, and I didn't care about myself.

I first studied psychology in high school. I somehow found myself in an advanced placement psychology class (the class the "smart kids" got into) and would drag myself there at seven in the morning after having woken up twenty minutes before, hanging outside of my boyfriend's car window looking down at a pile of my own vomit, thinking to myself, "I could have died last night." I was completely detached from how serious an issue almost dying is—drinking Jack and Coke on a stomach full of ecstasy and cheap takeout food doesn't usually end well.

I made it to college, only for the first few years' progress to look like moving from passing out dangling from cars to passing out underneath them. (I'm not sure which was safer; definitely neither.) At twenty-two years old, I was diagnosed with borderline personality disorder after a wild drug-fueled binge where I'm pretty sure I was roofied and, again, almost died. My whole life changed with this diagnosis. Borderline personality disorder, BPD for short, is a disorder characterized by unstable relationships, self-image, emotions, and behavior.[2] Impulsivity. Promiscuity. Suicidality. And a deep fear of being *out of control*. Bingo! In my early twenties, the label fit.

This, along with an ultimatum from my high school boyfriend (now husband), fueled a deep desire to change. It wasn't the blanket ultimatum he gave me, "Change or I'll leave you," that did it. It was that, when he said this, I heard, "Change, or you'll lose the greatest person in your life," and I didn't want that to happen. It was the first time I really took a look inward. The first time I allowed myself to say: **"For how much control you think you have over your life, you sure are fucking it up. Ready to stop?"** And I was.

Whether a new diagnosis, an ultimatum, a simple desire to better your life, or something else led you to this book, I'm glad you're here. This book is about change. It's about control. It's about choosing to work on yourself despite feeling afraid to do so. Despite feeling like all forces are working against you. And we're going to do this by looking at parts of you that are hidden. Parts of you that you may not know exist. Systems and functions that decide (more than you do, right now at least) what you think and feel and how you behave.

For decades, the psychology field shunned people with my BPD diagnosis. Therapists would actively choose not to work with people like me (and some still do). *"They are the way they are, and they always will be."* As terrible as this sounds, it makes sense. Human beings don't want to do hard shit, and helping someone change whose behavior patterns are deeply rooted in survival, anxiety, and fear *is* hard shit.

But look, it's not just people with mental (or physical) illnesses whose bodies, brains, and minds may be out of control. Most of our thoughts, feelings, and behaviors occur at the hands of our unconscious (the part of us that lies *outside* our awareness), meaning a lot of the time, we don't actually decide what to think or feel or how to behave. This may sound like a cop-out, but it's not. It's the *truth*.

Your unconscious is powerful—way more powerful than your consciousness (the part of you that you are aware of). The reason we get stuck with habits we wish we could change, behaviors that hurt ourselves and others, and thoughts and feelings we don't want is that our body, brain, and mind are unconsciously trying to protect us, unconsciously trying to keep us alive. For the unconscious, *survival, not happiness, is the goal.*

You likely define yourself by your conscious choices: By decisions "you" made, thoughts "you" had, and things "you" felt. The person you married, the job you applied for, the invitation you turned down. The thing is, though, almost all of these experiences take place unconsciously. Multiple theories have explored and tried to find the true relationship between our consciousness and our unconscious (how what we *are* aware of is influenced by what we're *not*), and on a fundamental level, they tend to agree on one thing: Your unconscious controls at least 95 percent of all of your thoughts, feelings, behaviors, and perspectives.[3] Yet, your consciousness takes most of the credit for it.

An article in *Time* magazine titled "Why You're Pretty Much Unconscious All the Time"[4] describes the relationship between your unconscious and your consciousness like this: The conscious "you" is like a not-so-smart CEO whose staff (all your unconscious parts) does all the work and all the research and then hands the CEO the documents to sign. The CEO signs and takes *all* the credit.

This is what I was doing for years with my own body, brain, and mind, except I thought it was cool to be the CEO of a company whose staff was fucking shit up all the time—it wasn't. And it's probably what

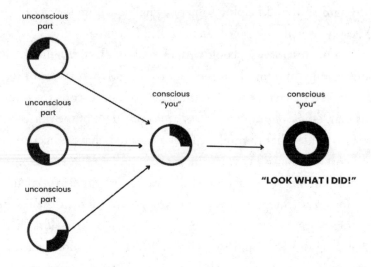

you're doing, too—taking credit, good or bad, for things your unconscious is doing.

You are the person most responsible for your life. And *you* are the greatest person in your life. You deserve to change for yourself. You deserve to give yourself the ultimatum you've been needing. You deserve to show yourself that this isn't just "the way you are" and the way "you'll always be."

A truth: As smart and as capable as we've become as a species, we're still wildly unconscious and out of control. Another truth: You can be in control of what's out of your control, and this book will teach you how to do that.

Some people say we don't need bitches in our lives. I can't entirely agree. Sometimes, they make life more interesting and more fun. And you know who the biggest bitch in your life is right now? Your unconscious. That bitch shows up everywhere, never leaves your side, wants full control, and doesn't make the best choices unless you've done a lot of work to put it in its place.

TRUTH TAKEAWAY: You don't need to get rid of your unconscious. You do need to learn how to control it.

The Serenity Prayer on Steroids

There's a universal law of control that influences you as a human being, one that can push you straight down a path toward your own demise if not understood properly. The Law of Control states that we feel good about ourselves to the degree to which we feel we are in control of our lives. Our control is our power; when we feel out of control, we often feel powerless.

In psychology, we refer to this concept as the *locus of control.*[5] Your "locus" is where you think control over the events in your life is located. You can either have an *internal* locus of control or an *external* locus of control. People who possess an internal locus of control believe that they hold the power to shape their own lives and that their actions have the potential to influence the outcomes they experience. Conversely, those with an external locus of control believe that factors beyond their influence play a majority, if not all, of the role in determining how their lives play out.

"IT'S ON ME"	"IT'S ON THEM"	"IT DEPENDS"
internal locus of control	external locus of control	mixed locus of control

Guess which locus of control is present in these situations: internal, external, or mixed?

Situation 1: You just took a test. You failed it. You studied, but not as much as you could have because "What does it matter anyway?" You see others receive passing grades. Now you're calling them "lucky" and the test "rigged." Rather than trying to improve your study methods or email your professor, you immediately drop the class.*

Situation 2: You hear that your company has an opening for a position you're qualified for. There's a lot of competition. You start to take initiative and tell yourself, "I'm going to try for this. Why not?" You

---

* External locus of control.

expand your skills, take on additional responsibilities, and network with colleagues (even though you hate it). You get the promotion.*

Situation 3: You're facing a complex problem. You feel overwhelmed and complain about external factors getting in your way. Yet, you're open to and ask for your colleagues' input, research potential solutions, and do your best because you believe that "you determine your future." The solutions don't work, and the issue remains. You review the internal and external causes of the failure and bring them to your boss. You're willing to keep trying.†

People who feel that outside forces control their life (like in Situation 1) often blame others and find it hard to get past tough times. Those who feel in charge of their own life (as in Situation 2) stay positive, handle good and bad times, and bounce back quickly. Some folks experience a mix of both (shown in Situation 3), switching between feeling in control and feeling controlled by outside forces.

What is *your* locus of control?

Start by asking yourself these four questions:[6] (Write them down, along with your answers. Take this shit seriously and it can change your life.)

1. Do I have a hard time saying "no" when someone tries to sell me something?
2. When I want something, do I work hard to get it?
3. When something is going to affect me, how much do I learn about it?
4. Do I feel like I have earned the good things that have happened to me?

The first question will give you insight into how quickly you release control of your decisions; the second and third, how much control you

---

* Internal locus of control.

† Mixed locus of control.

think you have; and the fourth, how much you believe your actions influence your outcomes.

If you feel like you don't have much control over things happening to you right now, this book is here to help you see that you can control more than you think, especially your own perspectives and decisions. I'm glad you're reading it. If you already feel like you have some control, we're off to a great start. And if the idea of control being in- or outside of you was new when you started reading, then I've done part of my work. You've gained awareness of something that was influencing your life without you knowing it—how whether you believe you're in control or not determines if you can be. You're aware of it (for now at least), and you can start using it to make a difference in your life.

One way to quickly start shifting control from outside of you to inside of you is to ask yourself, "What more can I do?" or "Could I have done something differently to get what I wanted?" whenever you're about to make a decision or after something happens. Then, try your best to do those extra things.

Now, there's a saying often spoken within the rooms of one of our country's most prominent self-help groups, Alcoholics Anonymous, that goes like this:

> "Grant me the serenity to accept the things I cannot change, the courage to change the things I can, and the wisdom to know the difference."*

It's called the serenity prayer;[7] it's changed the lives of millions of people, and it has lessons you could benefit from learning (regardless of whether you have substance use issues). Let's break it down line by line.

> "Grant me the serenity to accept the things I cannot change."

---

* I removed "God" from the breakdown because it's important the exercise is applicable to all people. I encourage you to adjust as desired.

Let's be honest. There are countless things we wish we could change—how quickly stoplights turn when we're running late, whom our ex married instead of us, and the difference in volume between our favorite TV shows and the loud-ass commercials that come on between acts—and we can't. At least not on our own. Yet, we allow ourselves to get absolutely livid at our inability to do so. I've certainly been caught yelling at a light pole at 7:58 a.m. on a Monday morning, blaming it for my tardiness.

Serenity means experiencing a sense of calm, tranquility, and peace of mind. It's about feeling free from stress, worries, and emotional chaos. Can you imagine being calm even when you're late? Content when someone you love is with "the wrong person"? Fine with adjusting the volume every five minutes? This book will teach you how to do that. It's not going to teach you how to become an emotionless zombie (who wants that?), but it will lead you to have more of a choice, more control, over how you think, feel, and respond to things in your life that you can't change.

"[Give me] the courage to change the things I can."

Now, courage is tricky. You can have it, even when you think you don't, if you change how you define and perceive it. When people think of courage, they often think of big feats like bungee jumping off a large bridge, proposing to the love of their life, or saying "yes" to a job in a new country. But courage is simply taking action, even when you feel afraid or uncertain. It doesn't have to be a monumental moment.

As humans, we're programmed to resist change and only to change if we *really* feel like it will help us survive. Your unconscious desires the path of least resistance. So perhaps it isn't that you're "not courageous." Perhaps it's that you're running on a blueprint that helped you survive during a time period you're no longer in, and it's time to tell yourself the time for change has come.

For something to be courageous, you need to label it as such. It was courageous for you to pick up this book. You have no idea what's in it, but you're spending your time on it. You took action, even when uncertain. Perhaps you're afraid to change, afraid to be in control of yourself, and still . . . here you are. The courage is there. Start recognizing it, and let's apply it to those more difficult situations, shall we?

"[Help me find] the wisdom to know the difference."

This book is basically the serenity prayer on steroids. It's going to help you gain the wisdom to know the difference between what you can and can't change and control when it comes to your body, brain, and mind through the lens of mental health and healing, through the lens of what you're consciously aware of at any given time and what lies outside your awareness—in your unconscious. This book will show you how to find the right mix of being okay with what you can't control and that which you can.

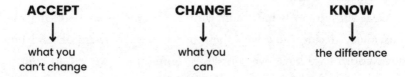

ACCEPT	**CHANGE**	**KNOW**
↓	↓	↓
what you can't change	what you can	the difference

There are aspects of life, circumstances, and events that are beyond your control, and we must acknowledge this from the get-go. In this book you're going to change your perceptions, your actions, and your decisions. What you can't immediately change using this book? The type of world you live in. One where some human beings aren't treated like humans at all. The final part of this book will teach you how to use what you've learned to make a positive impact on other people and your community. But first, you need to see how your unconscious shows and take specific steps (12 Steps, to be exact) toward your own healing so you can be as effective as possible in helping others in the future.

How Your Unconscious Is Showing

When asked to picture someone whose "unconscious is showing," people tend to imagine a person on the brink of a psychological break, acting in ways that make it clear they need serious help. Or, more mildly, someone who needs to be psychoanalyzed to see where all their trauma is stored.

> **KNOW YOUR TERMS:** Psychoanalyze: To examine someone's mind to understand their thoughts and behaviors.

While this can be the case for some individuals, your unconscious doesn't just show up as a result of trauma you've experienced. There's a lot more to it.

We all have unconscious thoughts, feelings, behaviors, and perceptions that aren't entirely healthy or beneficial to us or others, even if those unconscious parts of us are more socially acceptable or less socially visible than others. Just because we don't label something "out of control" doesn't mean it *can't* be. And just because something is "in our control" doesn't mean it *always* is.

We're *all* human beings built with an internal guidebook that unconsciously decides how we function, what we're aware of, and how much control we have over ourselves. Sometimes, we feel in control; other times, we don't. Sometimes we make conscious choices and live in the present moment; many other times, we find ourselves saying things like "I have no idea how I remembered to do that," or "How did I not feel that?" or "It's like I keep dating the same person over and over again, just in different bodies, by accident," or "I don't know why, but I'm getting weird fucking vibes from that person over there." *That.* That's your unconscious showing.

So the first question to ask isn't "*Is* your unconscious showing?" It is showing. The first question is: "*How* is your unconscious showing?" Let's briefly discuss the three parts of the unconscious and how they show up in you and your life to help you gain immediate awareness.

#1: Your body responds and reacts without your conscious awareness or control

This is your somatic unconscious. It's composed of things like somatic perception, physiological processes, nonverbal cues, and nervous system responses. Somatic perception is how you feel and experience body sensations—temperature, touch, movement, and that feeling you get when the person massaging you has absolutely no idea what they're doing. (. . . Pressure? No, pain? Either works.) Physiological processes include your heart changing pace, your breathing leveling out, and butterflies in your stomach. Nonverbal cues look like facial expressions that show your mood, slumped shoulders when you're experiencing sadness, and avoiding eye contact when you're lying. Nervous system responses include your fight-or-flight response and survival reflexes like pulling your hand off a hot stove.

You can, of course, be consciously aware of these things; however, you often only become aware of them *while* or *after* they're happening, meaning, typically, you don't consciously choose to slump your shoulders because you feel defeated, feel like you're going to vomit before a first date, or give away your dishonesty because you can't look into someone's eyes. It just happens.

The concept of your body being out of your control is typically familiar to people who experience chronic pain, physical disability, or illness; people recovering from surgery; and other similar conditions and situations. This isn't something new when thought of from a physical health or medical perspective. Thinking about it through the lens of mental health, however, has just begun booming in the last few decades.

The point here is that your body, in a way, has a mind of its own, and it's probably about time you started listening to it.

#2: Your brain thinks, perceives, judges, and interprets almost completely on its own

This is your cognitive unconscious. This part of your unconscious includes the mental processes and information that operate outside your conscious awareness. It involves behaviors like buying into stereotypes (cognitive misers), experiencing FOMO, or the "Fear of Missing Out" (primary evolutionary motives), automatically returning someone's smile (mimicry), and getting stressed when your partner is stressed (emotional contagion).

Your brain is lazy. It doesn't want to think any more than it has to. It's a cognitive miser, meaning it has a tendency to solve problems using the least amount of energy and effort possible. Got asked a question that could have multiple answers? Just give the first answer that pops into your head. This is the fastest way to be right! (*Your brain thinks a quicker answer is a better answer.*) See that blond girl over there? She's going to be just like the other ones. Don't talk to her. (*Your brain doesn't want to experience pain, and it generalizes to avoid doing so.*)

Primary motives mean that when it comes down to it, your brain will prioritize decisions you make by whether those decisions will help you survive, avoid disease, reproduce, and more—like unknowingly judging tanning or diet products more positively when you're looking for a partner than when you're not.[8] Your brain thinks, "Perhaps these things aren't that bad for me considering they seem to lead to a goal I have . . ." Your beliefs change depending on what's most important to both you *and* your unconscious brain.

Mimicry and contagion occur when you get mad when your partner's mad, when a child learns to cope with their emotions because they see their parent engage in regulation techniques, and when frontline workers experience what's known as vicarious trauma[9]—which is when the constant exposure to others' traumatic events cause professionals to experience traumatic symptoms themselves, like difficulty concentrating or having nightmares.

Again, of course, you can be aware of these things, but it's when your cognitive unconscious is running *without* your conscious awareness, without having some light shed onto its unknown processes, that things can get messy—like in instances of taking on abusive behaviors seen in your family or relationships, jumping too quickly to conclusions and missing out on great friendships or opportunities, or going against your values because you felt pressured or afraid (which is when your unconscious works best).

It can be scary to realize your brain learns about, judges, perceives, and interprets your life all on its own. But by the time you're done reading this book, you'll be damn happy it does because you'll be able to control its process in one or two ways: Either you'll learn to control and change the cognitive systems in your brain, or you'll learn to control whether or not you actually listen to the choices your brain is making. Ideally, you'll learn both.

#3: What you experience unconsciously affects how you feel about yourself, others, and the world

Finally, your psychoanalytic unconscious. This is probably the one you're most familiar with. Most self-help books refer to this as the "subconscious" and are referencing Sigmund Freud's idea of the unconscious when doing so. I don't like the word "subconscious." My belief is that the majority of the public jumped on board the generalized and pop-psych-infused concepts of Freud's theories, limiting many to stay focused on how our *mind* can get out of control, taking away attention and conscious awareness from how our physical *body* and *brain* cognition affect us, too. On top of that, Freud didn't use the word "subconscious" outside of a few early years of his career and yet, many of us still do (more on this in Chapter Two).

Try putting the word "subconscious" into Google Scholar. Ninety-eight percent of the articles will use the word "unconscious" in its place. Now, try searching "subconscious" using the regular version of Google. It's littered with pop articles, mostly containing bullshit information breaking down aspects of the subconscious for clicks.

The thing most people get wrong about the psychoanalytic unconscious is that they assume it's something controlled strictly by your psychological experiences. If you have new experiences, you'll change and feel better. And while this may be true, there are mechanisms of the mind that are automatic and default. They can't and won't change. Some of these mechanisms include counterfactuals, the pain–pleasure principle, and learned helplessness (which—spoiler—is a misnomer since it isn't really *learned* at all).

Counterfactuals are thoughts about what might have happened or what could have happened. They're when you say things like "If only

I didn't do that," and find yourself in a tornado of best-case scenarios that will never happen. This sounds like anxiety and regret, and it is. But it's the *automatic* part of it. The part you need to learn exists not just because you're psychologically upset with yourself or you have low self-esteem but because this is how you unconsciously function as a human being—no matter what you've been through.

The pain–pleasure principle applies to the fact that you, as a human, will always move *toward* pleasure and *away* from pain, naturally. It's not a function of your existence you can change. Instead, it's something you can come to understand and adjust, physiologically and conceptually.

Another aspect of your psychoanalytic unconscious, learned helplessness—when your life experiences eventually lead you to "give up" on yourself—is often seen as a moral failing, as an inability to be strong through adversity. The failure is on *us* as a society. Helplessness is not always conscious, but it is always potentially unconscious. When our brain truly thinks there's nothing it can do, it will tell us to stop trying or to not try at all. It doesn't mean it's right (because, remember, your brain is a cognitive miser), but it will certainly think it is.

Your job throughout the nine chapters of this book is to do the work, to uncover how your life experiences have created your psychoanalytic unconscious and hijacked your somatic and cognitive unconscious to create the automatic thoughts, feelings, perceptions, and decisions you make—and to do something about it.

I've just introduced you to The New Three-Part Unconscious: **the somatic, the cognitive, and the psychoanalytic.**

Your three-part unconscious, not just your "subconscious," is a powerful, messy, sometimes wrong, often risky, usually helpful to some degree, aspect of you. As human beings, that's something absolutely crucial you start to give a shit about. While you'll get to know exactly what each part does for you in the upcoming chapters, here's a one-line definition for each:

Your somatic unconscious: The *reactions* and *sensations* that occur within your body without your conscious awareness or control.

Your cognitive unconscious: The *perceptions* and *information processing* that occur within your brain without your conscious awareness or control.

Your psychoanalytic unconscious: The *experiential outcomes* that influence you without your conscious awareness or control.

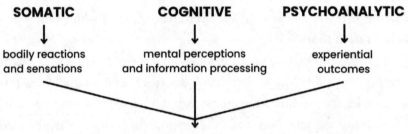

THE NEW THREE-PART UNCONSCIOUS

SOMATIC	COGNITIVE	PSYCHOANALYTIC
↓	↓	↓
bodily reactions and sensations	mental perceptions and information processing	experiential outcomes

occur without your conscious awareness or control

Before we dive into how to actively change your life with the steps I've outlined in the second part of this book, and before we go into detail about each part in Chapters Three to Five, I need to explain how these parts work together to steer the direction of your life. And, yes, I will, in the next section, be using a car analogy (original, I know).

Controlling the "Uncontrollable"

Think about a vehicle: its intended function, its parts, its driver, and the type of gas they choose to put in the car.

Okay . . . how does this all relate to your three-part unconscious?

Your somatic unconscious (comprised of your body and your brain) is like the car and its parts. Your arms and legs are like the four wheels of a car—they help you move and get from point A to point B. The inside of the car is like the inside of your body—you can take care of it or, like many of us, struggle to feel comfortable even thinking about it because . . . well, it's a disaster in there. And the engine is like your brain—without it, you simply wouldn't work.

Like the body of a car, if we lack an understanding of how to operate our own physical body and don't learn what it feels like to have our bodies running smoothly, not only will we show up in an overwhelmed, discombobulated, uncoordinated manner (much like a student driver, or just an overall terrible one, does), but it can also impact how comfortable we feel on this ride called life. It's sort of like when your vehicle has the option to smooth out the bumpiness of the road, and you don't find out about it until you've had the car for a year, wondering to yourself, "Why didn't I just read the manual? I've been frustrated this whole time when I didn't need to be."

Your cognitive unconscious involves how the engine (or your brain) *operates*. Neurodiversity, a term used to describe the non-pathological differences in how the human brain controls thing like movement, sociability, learning and attention, and other mental functions,[10] is represented well when thinking about how different car engines function—some automatic, some manual, some adjustable. Some are maximized for certain tasks, and some can't complete certain tasks without significant conscious control and effort, if at all.

When it comes to how our brain's cognition works, imagine putting a car into self-driving mode. To some, it's a blessing. To others, a curse. Tesla's new self-driving mode, for example, is one of my own personal nightmares. It seems (at least for me) that "automatic" mode means the car will see green lights when they're red, see red lights when they're green, will decide to mess around in the fast lane until I have 0.2 miles left to exit the freeway, and will mimic the driving pace of the car in front of me when I'm late to an important meeting. Just like Tesla's self-driving mode, your unconscious doesn't give a fuck what your goals are; it will only do what it's programmed to do unless you tell it otherwise.*

---

* Elon, I know you've made improvements. We all start somewhere, just like my readers. Progress, not perfection. Don't sue me.

Lastly, your psychoanalytic unconscious is like the driver and the type of gas that gets put in the car. Sometimes you decide where to drive the car, and sometimes you put the gas in. Other times, other people have control over where you're headed (they're in the driver's seat), and sometimes they put in the wrong type of gas, the kind that just fucks your car up completely.

Your psychoanalytic unconscious involves the experiences you have in your life and how they begin to have an automatic, and often unknown, effect on you and your behavior. So, for example, as much as this does absolutely no justice to the feelings and outcomes associated with abuse and neglect, someone enacting traumatic violence onto you is similar to someone putting diesel in your non-diesel car. What you experience in life can either help you function efficiently and with ease, or it can cause you to seize up, clog your internal ability to function, and completely and utterly break you down.

The ways you drive your car, whom you let drive your car, and the type of gas you put in your car are like deciding the type of experiences you want to have and the places you want to go in your life. The upsetting part? Just like we're only allowed to be passengers in a car for around the first fifteen years of our lives, we're usually passengers of our life experiences until we're afforded the time, space, agency, and opportunity to decide for ourselves. Many of us still lack full agency and opportunity well into adulthood, for both internal and external, conscious and unconscious reasons—like when we're held back by our own or others' decisions, and, at times, aren't even aware it's happening.

> **TRUTH TAKEAWAY:** Just like a car, your body and brain work best when you take good care of them and understand how they work from the inside out.

Switching gears (pun intended), let's talk about a concept I briefly described above: the ability for a car to run manually, automatically, or both ways.

The important part of this analogy is that even when you put the car in automatic, you're deciding when to do so and your final destination. Either you can put it into self-driving mode (with the correct address, hopefully) and sit back and chill, or if you don't have that option, you can put it on cruise control until you need to put your foot back on the gas to ensure you stop at your intended location. Different brains and different bodies come equipped with varying options.

As humans, we are not just manual nor are we fully automatic. We are a mixed bag of greatness, sort of like a hybrid. We are consciousness and unconsciousness mixed into a glorious organic vehicle that can either drive us up the mountains of our greatest dreams or down into the depths of a ditch, almost killing us (sort of like that one time my dad drove his car off a cliff while on psychedelic mushrooms—but I digress).

Similar to how drivers can switch between manual and automatic, humans can shift between conscious and unconscious behavior depending on the situation. Sometimes, conscious control is necessary, requiring you to actively engage and make deliberate choices. Other times, unconscious processes take over, guiding your actions based on previous learning and automatic responses. The control doesn't lie in whether or not you're in manual or automatic. It lies in whether you're in control of *when* the mode switches, how, why, and what happens next.

It's not that the unconscious parts of you we're talking about in this book are uncontrollable. It's that they function in a certain way, and you need to learn what those ways are in order to control them as best you can.

It's not: Is this aspect of you as a human conscious or unconscious?

It is: How does this part of you work when it's unconscious, and then, can you consciously do something to change and control it when you want to?

Striving for a balanced approach—knowing when to consciously engage and when to allow unconscious processes to take the wheel—can lead to greater self-awareness, personal growth, and more adaptive responses to life's challenges.

When you walk into a room, instantly feel your heart pounding, your skin sweating, and notice your brain saying, "Leave. Leave now.

This was a bad idea," you deserve to be able to pause and control how you consciously respond. Is this *really* a bad idea, or is this situation just *unfamiliar* to your body, brain, and mind? Is your automatic analysis of the situation one you *want* to react to or one you'd like to ignore and push through? *You* should control the next step, not your unconscious.

When you instantly fall for someone because they're your "type," you deserve to pause and truly ask yourself, "Is this person my 'type' or my unconscious '*pattern*'? Is this the easier way out of loneliness, according to my unconscious, or am I *actually* safe to continue bonding with this person because I've consciously assessed both my needs and what I can give at this time to a relationship?"

When I say this book will help you gain control, I don't mean controlling your unconscious like taming some wild beast (not like I like the sound of that, anyway). I mean you'll be able to use your consciousness to control and change whether or not you listen to your unconscious and, at times, what your unconscious does in the first place.

UNCONSCIOUS BEHAVIOR	CONSCIOUS BEHAVIOR
~95%	~5%
automatic	manual
faster	slower
stronger	weaker
stubborn	yielding
dominant	submissive

Why Should I Care That My Unconscious Is Showing?

As difficult as it can be to admit you're not as conscious as you'd like, your unconscious is an easy thing to see "showing" once you start looking for it. Knowing and accepting it's showing is the first stage of growth. Caring about the impact it's having on your life is the second.

If you don't care about your unconscious and how and when it shows, you're basically not giving a shit about 95 percent of yourself. Doesn't sound very good, does it? Caring about your unconscious parts is the only way to truly become the person you want to be. It's how you consciously change the way you feel, think, and act in life. And as you can tell from my point regarding learned helplessness and the psycho-analytic unconscious, it's a dangerous thing to ignore—it can tell you to give up, sometimes on your life completely. If you don't understand what's happening, you can succumb to its hopelessness.

The moment we make the decision to control our lives consciously, we immediately enter into a face-to-face battle with our unconscious—who doesn't want to lose and will do almost anything not to change. Your unconscious has been forming within you since before you were born. It's extremely strong, deeply rooted, and very afraid. Your con-sciousness, on the other hand, takes work, not only to develop but to maintain. It's weaker (by design, not default) and easily hands the reins over to your unconscious whenever it isn't sure, isn't present, or isn't im-mediately capable of controlling the situation.

The most difficult part about knowing your unconscious is showing? Making the choice to look at it, intensely, and begin consciously con-trolling it—because, yes, it can be done; and you should certainly get started today.

If you're like me and just about everyone else I know, you've spent most of your life running on autopilot, doing, feeling, thinking, and perceiving the same things, the same way, over and over again, despite your best intentions to perceive, think, feel, and do otherwise. You may be stuck thinking the same negative thoughts about yourself and other people or engaging in the same shitty behaviors you know aren't good for you, your relationships, your productivity, or your path forward.

We're at a place in our lives where we're spending more time keeping up with the Joneses or the Kardashians than keeping up with how our own bodies function. We think more about which ketchup to buy at the store when our usual brand is out of stock and more time thinking about what other people think about us than how and why we're having thoughts in our own heads to begin with. And we're blaming ourselves for simply being human. For experiencing different levels of sensitivity than those around us, wanting to move toward things that make us feel better instead of worse (even if that means our to-do list doesn't get done), and succumbing, for example, to the "I can't control this or me or anything" thought that develops as an evolutionary benefit for our lazy-ass brain. It's time to recover from being human. Not because there's something wrong with being human, but because no one taught us how to do it in the first place.

Just as I was a bitch—you know, overly aggressive and wildly unpleasant—before I was a therapist, we're all unconscious before we're conscious. And just as I can still be a bitch sometimes, we're all still unconscious at times. The goal of this book is not to teach you how to be perfect or how to be conscious of everything all the time (that's not even possible). It cannot guide you on how to completely change the unchangeable or control the uncontrollable.

What this book will teach you is how to consciously change your unconscious and how to control the uncontrollable—*just enough to change your life*.

You can consciously control what you care about.

Will you care about *you*?

CHAPTER 1 SUMMARY

- The more in control you feel, the more powerful you feel.
- There's a lot more than the "subconscious" controlling you without you knowing.
- Your somatic unconscious is all the things your body does automatically.
- Your cognitive unconscious involves how your brain can be lazy, biased, and manipulated.
- Your psychoanalytic unconscious develops from your life experiences.
- Human behavior can be conscious (like driving a manual car) and unconscious (like cruising in automatic); the power comes from controlling when you switch gears.

2

You're Thinking About It All Wrong

Imagine you're in a darkened warehouse; it's totally pitch-black.

In this warehouse is everything you need to live your life and understand yourself—instruments to measure your bodily needs like hydration and blood pressure, categorical lists of comparisons (safe or unsafe, lucky or unlucky, important or not important), and photos and videos of your least and most favorite people, places, and experiences.

You can't see anything in the warehouse. But in your hand, you hold a small yet powerful flashlight you can use to navigate through the darkness. The only parts of the warehouse you can see at any given time are what you see with the beam of the flashlight. The warehouse is your three-part unconscious. The flashlight is your consciousness.

In her book *Dying to Be Me*,[1] Anita Moorjani describes a near-death experience she had in 2012 as her internal warehouse becoming completely lit up—and changing her life forever.

> **KNOW YOUR TERMS:** Near-Death Experience: A profound psychological event that may occur to someone close to death or in extreme physical or emotional crisis.

Imagine that one day, big floodlights go on, so the whole warehouse is illuminated, and you realize it's huge and lined with shelves and shelves of all kinds of different things. Every kind of thing you can imagine, and ones you can't even imagine, all exist on these shelves.

Some are beautiful; some not so beautiful. Some large, some small. Some things in colors you've never seen before, colors you've never imagined to exist. You've seen some of them before with your flashlight, but many of them you've never laid eyes on because your flashlight has never shone on them.

Now, imagine the lights go off again. Although all you can see is what's being shown in the beam of your one flashlight, you now know there is so much more that exists simultaneously and alongside (not beneath) the things that you can see.[2]

According to Anita, as she was close to dying, she suddenly saw all the hidden parts of herself, like a huge, dark room lighting up and revealing everything inside—she had gained conscious awareness of her entire unconscious. Knowledge and insight flooded in, like turning on the lights in a vast storage space. But this metaphor doesn't just pertain to near-death experiences.

You have a flashlight within you right now—your consciousness.

Your flashlight is likely shining outward at this very moment—onto the pages of this book, the scene or objects you're currently looking at, or the faces of the people around you. It's taking in written words or spoken sounds and giving them to your unconscious, which then processes

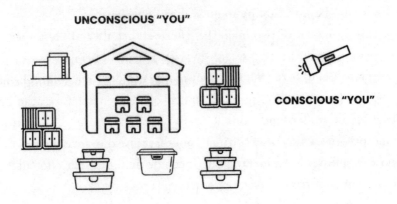

UNCONSCIOUS "YOU"

CONSCIOUS "YOU"

them and returns to you an understanding of what's being said. You're "reading," and you *know* you are.

You don't need to wait for a life-threatening situation to have a transformative conscious experience. You also don't need to have a non-near-death "floodlight" experience by, for example, dropping a bunch of acid or taking an Ayahuasca journey to spiritually delve into your unconscious, either. You could; it would probably be faster, but I can't recommend it.[3] You do, however, at minimum, need to make a conscious choice to gain the insight needed—to know what's in your warehouse and to know it well.

> **MAKE IT SIMPLE:** You don't need extreme experiences to explore your unconscious. Your consciousness, although limited, gives you direct and personal access to it at all times.

Speaking of spiritual and drug-induced experiences leading to a heightened level of consciousness, this is where so many limit themselves. People think they need to grow their hair down to the floor, develop an obsession with crystals, and get a peace sign tattoo in the middle of their forehead to be a "conscious" person.[4] In other words, they think that in order to like, use, or understand consciousness, they need to become a hippie.

Don't get me wrong, I love hippies and hippie-type people. Some of the people who have changed my life for the better could likely be categorized under the umbrella of "hippie." But, it's not just this type of people who have the ability to grow their consciousness.

This is one out of two major belief errors that are actively impeding many of our abilities to consciously grow as human beings.

Human Belief Error #1: Consciousness is solely a spiritual concept.

We've been attempting to get much of the general American civilization to understand consciousness through the lens of spiritual concepts—it's a woo-woo spiritual tool that is used to help you become more enlightened. And okay, yeah, it can be that. But that's not all it is. That's not all it has to be.

Your consciousness *is* a tool, but it's more of an internal flashlight than a mystical telescope. You don't have to use it as a means to see the stars; you can instead use it as a way to explore the universe that's already within you. Consider me and your consciousness your psychedelic drugs, taking you on your own internal and environmental trip—one that will, hopefully, change your perspective in a way similar to (perhaps not quite as intense as) Anita's near-death experience.*

I briefly alluded to the second major belief error in Chapter One. Here it is:

Human Belief Error #2: The unconscious is solely a bad thing.

Modern-day theories about what drives behavior differ from those originally put forth by Sigmund Freud. This is partly because, while Freud was a neurologist, he didn't have access to the type of scientific inquiry and research tools we have today. Moreover, as stated in *Scientific American*, we've moved significantly beyond only studying people who would fall under the category of "abnormal" to looking at average groups of individuals and how we function on a fundamental level, not just when we're "disordered."[5]

When it comes to looking at consciousness and the unconscious in the twenty-first century, many researchers are taking the stance that our internal world is one *fully connected* that can operate in both conscious and unconscious mode. Moving further away from Freud's theories, which seemed to state that our unconscious was guided by a separate set of rules than those that drive our consciousness.[6] It's not. All of your parts are intertwined, mostly working in conjunction with one another to get things done.

Your unconscious is not just the lost and torn childhood memories in your mind. It is that, and it's so much more, too. As I've said, you don't need to eliminate your unconscious. It's not a "bad" thing. It's actually one of the most helpful things you have going for yourself as a human being.

Think about it.

---

* Eh, that was a little bold, but I left it.

Picture walking on a crosswalk. You see someone crossing opposite you, and there's a car headed straight for them. You suddenly scream without thinking about it. The person looks to their left, sees the car, and jumps out of the way. At that moment, you (and the other crosswalker) are *thanking* your unconscious for saving their life. But then, in the next moment, when you arrive at the wedding you were headed to, you think you see a mouse, suddenly scream (again without thinking), and end up scaring the caterer, who jumps and drops your best friend's wedding cake thirty minutes before the ceremony begins. You didn't consciously choose to do *that*, either. Both screams were unconscious. But now you're *blaming* yourself (and so is your best friend) for one of your actions.

The difference? You feel bad and want to do something about one of them: the one where someone got hurt (not saved) by your brain unconsciously thinking there was danger. And . . . you can. Doing something about your unconscious starts with realizing that it's changeable. It's malleable. It can work in your favor.

Consciousness allows you to control your unconscious to the degree that (1) you're able to, and (2) you put in the effort to. Your unconscious is not inherently bad. It's wired to do whatever it needs to do to protect you. The thing is, with the way our lives tend to go these days, we rarely decide *how* it should function and learn *why* it does what it does until it's gotten us into trouble. Until you have to pick up a self-help book and learn how to recover from being a human with a three-part unconscious. Until you lose your job because you were late again. Until you scream in the hallway of your best friend's wedding and feel like you ruined their special day.

TRUTH TAKEAWAY: Your unconscious is morally neutral, and consciousness isn't just some fluffy concept; it's the driver of intention.

It must be said that consciousness itself is not easy to define. It's a phenomenon that baffles us as human beings and has led us to encounter several problems—some easy, some hard. The "easy" problems to solve when it comes to consciousness are those around how it works: how we can report our own moods, focus our attention on certain things (or not), and deliberately control our own behavior.[7] The "hard problem"[8] when it comes to consciousness? The fact that we only *personally* experience it. The fact that you experience, but cannot share with a single other human being, the *exact* way the difference between sour and sweet tastes to you, the *exact* feeling of the vibrations of your favorite song played in real time at a concert, or your *personal* experience of being in a flow state—a state of complete immersion in an activity to the point where your sense of time is changed[9]—like reading a book from start to finish in one sitting or being "in the zone" during a sporting match.

We all experience consciousness, but we can't actually explain our experience to another person. It's too hard to. Why? Because no one *is* us except *us*.

As John Green, the author of one of the best-selling books of all time, *The Fault in Our Stars*, once wrote:

> "Consciousness is so weird. You have an interior life that is exclusively yours. It is as vast and as strange as my own interior life, but you can't really know mine, and I can't really know yours. Sometimes, seemingly out of nowhere, you remember that guy from high school who never wore pants, only shorts—no matter how cold it got. Being alive is just so, so weird."*

"Consciousness is so weird."
—John Green

We can put words to the conscious experience of our life events, but we can't ever actually share our experience, our *consciousness*, with other people.

While our understanding of the unconscious has been muddled by

---

* It is highly likely that John will delete this Thread at some point. It's just his thing. He wrote it; I promise.

the constant "subconscious, repressed" rhetoric, leading to a misunderstanding of how and why we function automatically as human beings, the concept of consciousness can often be a more difficult one to grasp. The way I see it: Most people accept that there are automatic (unconscious) parts of themselves, but they have a hard time realizing they can do something about it (use consciousness) without having to get into things like the spiritual world if they don't want to.

Let's define consciousness using the definition created by Antonio Damasio,[11] a neuroscientist who, as of writing this, is the chair of neuroscience at the University of Southern California, my alma mater:

Consciousness is the feeling and knowing of what happens. It's *you* being aware of your body and brain's reaction to the world and *knowing* your response to that experience.

For this book, you don't need to fully understand consciousness (no one does—not even the researchers who've dedicated their lives to studying it). What you need to know is that it exists within you, it's real, and it's the tool you can use (along with your unconscious) to change and control your life.

Having both conscious and unconscious parts of yourself makes you stronger and more capable of doing the things you love and the things that simply help you function on a daily basis. Just ask any person recovering from a stroke or another medical situation where they lost the ability to do basic tasks without consciously thinking about them—like walking, talking, or writing. These individuals can get better by *conscious choice*—by choosing to teach or reteach their body, brain, and mind new ways to think, feel, behave, and perceive themselves and their lives. They are activating an internal locus of control and changing their lives for the better.

They're choosing to consciously control and change their unconscious.

Eventually, if it's possible and they work hard enough at it, some parts of themselves will have them walking, talking, and writing *unconsciously* so other parts can learn to dance, sing, and draw *consciously*. The synergy you can create when your consciousness and unconscious work together is magic—like being able to identify when you're in unconscious sensory overload (and then consciously regulate yourself before overreacting) or when you adjust your automatic judgments of others to be judgments you can consciously trust even when they occur unconsciously—like, for example, thinking, "This is an unknown person to me, react carefully" instead of "This person is absolutely a bad person, judge negatively no matter what."

> **MAKE IT SIMPLE:** Consciously controlling your unconscious is teaching yourself how to do things without having to think about them.

All Your Parts

Let me tell you a story called "The Blind Men and the Elephant."[12]

Once upon a time, in a village in India, there lived six older men. Each was born blind. The local villagers loved and protected them, and travelers who crossed their paths would tell them stories about the world since they couldn't see it themselves.

Among all the stories, one thing intrigued them the most: elephants.

People told them that elephants could wreck forests, carry heavy loads, and scare everyone with their loud trumpet calls. But here's why they were so curious: They also knew that the rajah (the king) had a daughter who fearlessly rode these supposedly dangerous creatures. This left them wondering: Why would the rajah let his daughter anywhere near such scary beasts?

So, they started arguing about it. Day and night, they debated relentlessly, each stubbornly clinging to their *version of the truth*, each pulling the rope in their own direction—like a game of perceptual tug-of-war.

The first blind man proclaimed, "Elephants must be powerful creatures." He believed them to be colossal giants based on the stories he'd heard.

The second blind man, however, saw elephants as graceful and gentle creatures, saying that "if a princess rides on an elephant, this must be the case."

The third blind man insisted that elephants were deadly, stating, "You're wrong! I've heard that an elephant can pierce a man's heart with its horns."

The fourth blind man, skeptical and suspicious, dismissed the exaggerated tales. He responded by basically saying everyone was full of shit and that elephants were simply oversize cows.

The fifth blind man assumed elephants to be magical beings, thinking this could perhaps explain the princess's safe journeys even though elephants were "known to harm."

And the sixth blind man? Well, he just flat-out said they didn't exist. To him, it was simply impossible, and they were being pranked.

Each man based their version of the truth on the stories they'd been told, along with the best logical (and seemingly emotional) reasoning they could come up with.

The villagers got sick of their arguing and decided to put an end to it. They led the blind men to the rajah's grand palace to find out the truth about elephants once and for all.

When they arrived at the palace, a friend guided them to the courtyard where an elephant stood. Each man felt the elephant and shared his observations.

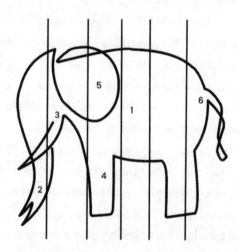

The first blind man touched the elephant's side and said, "An elephant is smooth and strong like a wall. It must be powerful." The second blind man, holding the trunk, announced, "No, an elephant is like a large snake, agile and flexible." The third blind man was examining one of the tusks when he said, "I knew it! This creature is sharp and deadly." The fourth blind man touched the elephant's leg and confidently asserted, "You guys are idiots. It's like I said . . . just a large cow." The fifth blind man was holding the elephant's ear. "An elephant is a mystical carpet that flies over mountains!" he shouted. And the sixth blind man grabbed the tail and called the elephant a worthless piece of rope.

They started getting pissed off at each other over this elephant, so pissed that their friend told them to go sit under a tree. (This was around the time of Buddha gaining enlightenment under trees, so it only made sense.) They went to the tree, but they kept at it. "Walls!" "Snake!" "Spear!" "No, cow!" "Carpet!" "Rope."

The rajah stopped the chaos by saying, "Enough!" (making it known he owned the place). He asked, "How can each of you be so certain you hold the absolute truth?" The blind men didn't know what to say, so the rajah continued:

"You have touched only parts of the elephant, my friends. *Perhaps, if you assemble the parts, you will begin to grasp the truth."*

Then the rajah told them to get the fuck out. The blind men returned to the village and began engaging in deep conversations along the journey back. Taking the rajah's advice, they shared their diverse experiences, seeking to assemble each of their separate truths. The blind men came to see there were flaws in their limited perspectives. They realized they needed to connect their experiences and insights to understand the elephant's true essence.

Each man was wrong, and each man was right. It isn't easy to come to the understanding of something as unique as an elephant if you aren't able to actually see it. This is the case with both your unconscious and your consciousness as well. They're unique to you; you can't *actually* see either of them (only their outcomes), and we've been fighting over each of their fundamental definitions for at least as long as we've been able to record our thoughts—shout-out to Descartes,[13] Locke,[14] and Nietzsche.[15]

According to Dr. Michael Craig Miller, in the Harvard Health blog, for more than a century, the general population has used the word "subconscious" to describe the reasoning behind their automatic, "beneath the surface" thoughts, feelings, behaviors, and perspectives.[16] This is limiting. It's us acting like the blind men, only touching one part of the true unconscious and deciding that's all we need to know. And in terms of consciousness, in the comment section of John's 2023 Thread about the guy who only wore shorts, spirituality was, of course, mentioned in the replies: "To me, you've just described spirituality."[17] Again, spirituality involves (and, I'd argue, requires) consciousness, but consciousness does not need to directly involve (and does not require) spirituality.

By eliminating the two human belief errors from your mind and accurately grasping the functionality of *all* your parts, you can reach a more complete understanding of the complex world that lives within you, start shifting your locus of control, and begin controlling your life.

I call my three-part unconscious "new" for two reasons.

First, there are at least two other "three-part" psychological theories related to the unconscious: Freud's three-part unconscious mind and Freud's three-part personality theory. The first involves the conscious, the "pre"-conscious, and the unconscious.[18] The second involves the id, superego, and ego.[19] These are all terms we'll revisit in Chapter Five.

Second, if you're not familiar with or are struggling to grasp the idea of my new three-part unconscious, it's likely not because the parts don't exist—each "part" has scientific evidence and entire fields of study dedicated to it—it's probably that you haven't seen it conceptualized the way I am doing for you now. It's not new information; it's a new perspective.

You've likely heard of the "mind–body" connection—the idea that our mind and body are inextricably linked—and that your body and brain want to do everything they can to keep you alive. What's less obvious to most people is how these three unconscious parts control our lives and make decisions for us without our awareness, and that clinicians and practitioners have been treating our three-part unconscious (mostly separately) for centuries.

While the term "somatic unconscious" isn't commonly or consistently used, there are many people who are already engaged in activating, changing, and controlling it. Many clinicians practice forms of psycho-therapy known as somatic therapies, including somatic experiencing and sensorimotor psychotherapy.

> **KNOW YOUR TERMS:** "Soma" means body in Greek. Somatic therapies are focused on the connection between mind and physical body experiences.

Somatic experiencing (SE) is a form of psychotherapy that works by having clients consciously witness the somatic perceptions associ-ated with certain, often traumatic, life experiences.[20] If you've ever heard someone talk about a therapy session where they brought up something difficult and then felt the sensations that came up in their body (and sat uncomfortably through it), it's likely some form of somatic experienc-ing. Sensorimotor psychotherapy is a body-centered form of traditional talk therapy that works similarly.[21]

An example of body-centric work outside (and within) the mental health field is biofeedback,[22] a therapy that uses special sensors attached to your body to teach you how to control physical functions, such as your heart rate, muscle tension, and sweating, which can help manage conditions like high blood pressure and chronic pain. Other activities that help the body's unconscious healing include yoga, acupuncture, and massage.

Your somatic unconscious isn't only listening when something is going terribly wrong. The body keeps the score, yes, not just of your traumas but of *everything* you experience in life. You need to remember this.

As for the "cognitive unconscious,"[23] this term exists in fields like psy-chology and neuroscience, with many therapies leveraging the idea that your brain is mostly automatic, including acceptance and commitment therapy (ACT)—a form of cognitive behavioral therapy shown to be helpful for many conditions, including for people who experience intense and intrusive thoughts due to obsessive-compulsive disorder (OCD).[24] Intrusive thoughts are strange, disturbing thoughts or images that seem to pop up in your mind out of nowhere.[25] ACT encourages acceptance of thoughts that come automatically to your mind and working on changing both how you relate to your thoughts and your behaviors in response to them.

In addition to cognitive psychotherapy, there are techniques like those used by occupational therapists to boost skills in focusing, remembering, planning, and solving problems. Thinking and decision-making are important not just for mental health issues but all the time, as your brain shapes *all* of what you do and think. In Chapter Four, we'll explore how these unseen mental processes affect your thoughts, which will be both enlightening and fun.

Lastly, the term "psychoanalytic unconscious" is often used as a synonym for the "unconscious mind." "Psychoanalytic" relates to the practice of psychoanalysis, a psychological method again originating from the infamous Sigmund Freud. Psychoanalysis is a form of therapy that attempts to access someone's unconscious mind in order to treat the mental health conditions they're experiencing.[26] Other forms of psychoanalytic-type therapy and treatment include psychodynamic psychotherapy—which is meant to help clients expand their self-awareness through understanding the influence of their past on their present behavior[27]—and self-psychology, a type of treatment based on the idea that you develop a sense of self that is grounded specifically in your past personal experiences, and that self-esteem comes from these experiences directly.[28]

Much of the discourse around the psychoanalytic unconscious, at least when it comes to conversations between friends or, these days, in "therapy-speak" news articles, is about how we function through a dysfunctional mind—one that makes us act like "narcissists" and "crazy people" and that tells us we're failing in romantic relationships because we had a bad relationship with our parents. These things can sometimes be true and should be addressed if need be. In addition to that, however, our psychoanalytic unconscious works in many ways that are unchangeable and that we shouldn't want to change: Ways that work for us but that we need to be careful with. Ways that we can leverage to keep ourselves in control, calmer, more confident, and more secure.

Every human is born relatively unconscious, with an internal environment that functions automatically and instinctually independent of instruction. Some researchers argue that babies are more conscious than adults are,[29] many have discussed how and when it actually develops[30] (pre-birth or in toddlerhood . . . etc.), and most of us are sitting here trying to figure out how we can become more conscious regardless of when we were first able to because, right now, our unconscious has much more of a hold on us than we'd like it to, and it's showing.

TRUTH TAKEAWAY: The three-part unconscious isn't just theory; it's real. Even though you can't see it, its signs and symptoms are exactly what healthcare pros look for when treating you (and not just the mental health ones).

The Real Human "Superpower"

In a world increasingly open to embracing and discussing mental health, it's not uncommon to come across statements referencing mental illnesses or conditions and traumatic experiences as superpowers.[31] Phrases like "ADHD is your superpower" or "Your trauma made you stronger" have gained traction, often well intentioned but frequently oversimplifying the complexities of mental health.

Unless nuanced and carefully presented, these phrases can sound like bullshit to a lot of people. Invalidating, even. To many, these assertions are dismissive, and for good reason—who wants to be told that experiencing debilitating anxiety or depression or going through a horrific violent attack is something to be proud of or thankful for?

The reality is that mental illness, mental disorders, trauma, and, unfortunately, even neurodivergent mental conditions can lead to worsened health outcomes, more life-functioning difficulties, and shortened lifespans. They absolutely are *not* superpowers . . . on their own.

The way I want you to think about mental disorders moving forward is that they are the unconscious out of control (this is likely a perspective you already had) and that every evidenced-based non-pharmaceutical intervention, including all named earlier in this chapter, use consciousness as the real human "superpower"—the one that allows you to become aware of, change, and control symptoms of things such as ADHD and trauma.

I think we can agree that Superman's ability to fly and Wonder Woman's ability to teleport* are only useful, only "superpowers," because they had *control* over them. I doubt we'd call either of them superheroes if all Superman could do was fly and crash into the middle of kids' birthday parties, breaking all their new toys, and all Wonder Woman could do was teleport into currently occupied porta-potties. It's because of the fact they can consciously decide when, how, why, and where to use these skills that they can save the world.

In my opinion, the only real superpower you will ever have when it comes to your mental health is the relationship between your unconscious and your consciousness.

"The only real superpower you will ever have . . . is the relationship between your unconscious and your consciousness."
—Dr. Courtney Tracy

Your unconscious helps you survive using your past and a prediction of your future. Your consciousness allows you to thrive (and fight) using in-the-moment awareness, decision-making, and control. Quoting Jazz Thornton,[32] a powerful advocate for mental health, it's time to

---

* Yes, Wonder Woman could teleport in the comics.

"stop surviving and start fighting." It's not what happened to you or the abilities you were born with or without that make you powerful. It's about what you do with it all. It's about shifting from passive survival, which is often governed by unconscious patterns and reactions (whether you have a mental illness or not), to active engagement and conscious control.

The stronger your unconscious is (and it's probably pretty strong), the harder you're going to have to work to control it. Not all parts are controllable or changeable—you have to breathe, your heart has to beat, you need to feel pain and get scared at times for your own safety, and you need to be able to make quick environment checks. But much of this can either be changed or controlled to work to your advantage.

The struggle to compete with your unconscious is universal. Individuals contending with chronic pain, autoimmune disorders, substance use disorders, mental health issues, or neuro-developmental challenges grapple with this daily. Yet, this challenge is not exclusive to them; it extends to habitual patterns and everyday thoughts and feelings, defining all of our behaviors, thoughts, interactions, and environment.

Someone who doesn't want to yell at their partner may find themselves yelling. A person who doesn't want to drink ever again may find themselves sitting at a bar after a difficult (or very exciting) day. A friend may judge a new colleague before actually getting to know them, even though their therapist told them to be open to meeting new people.

Although it's certainly a battle to harness your unconscious and change your life, complete consciousness isn't the ultimate goal. The ultimate goal is cultivating what I like to call a *consciously curated unconscious*. This involves building a rapport with your unconscious, understanding it, molding it, taking responsibility when it shows, and thanking it for existing because it's mostly what's keeping you alive. A consciously curated unconscious is an unconscious that is actively understood, intentionally molded, and held consciously responsible.

As you embark on this journey, consider the locus of control—the belief that you have the ability to influence the outcomes of your life. By embracing the relationship between your unconscious and consciousness as your true superpower, and by nurturing a consciously curated three-part unconscious, you can reclaim the driver's seat of your existence. You can finally turn on the flashlight and begin to look through, rearrange, and restructure your darkened warehouse.

You can start to care for yourself in a new way, in a new light.

CHAPTER 2 SUMMARY

- Don't wait until the end of your life to "see" yourself. You can start today.
- Consciousness isn't only a spiritual concept.
- Your unconscious isn't inherently bad.
- You're responsible for all your actions, whether you mean to do them or not.
- The only superpower you'll ever have is the relationship between your unconscious and your consciousness.
- You don't need to get rid of your unconscious; you need to understand and control it.

3

What You Feel Is What You Think

The Somatic Unconscious

"I don't want to feel this way."

When you work in behavioral health treatment, you hear this phrase repeated over and over again by different people, in different tones, for different reasons. It's an outward message or inner thought that emphasizes the difficulty of being in a conscious human body when that body is experiencing a sensation we'd rather avoid.

For some of us, one of the biggest upsets of being alive is that we have the ability to feel. Sure, orgasmically peaking with a partner in the bedroom may make us scream "Fuuuuck," but so can stubbing our pinky toe on the corner of our couch. Notably, however, the former likely ends in a "yes!" while the latter tends to end with a "no!"

As humans, we feel, and we aren't always happy about it.

In the fall of 2015, the three clients sitting in my group therapy session were certainly not happy about their ability to feel. At the time, I was a budding twenty-four-year-old clinician obtaining my master's degree,[1] working at a Malibu addiction rehab facility. I had made the decision a few months prior to "work with what's in the room"—meaning instead of structuring my groups around a predetermined therapy skill or theme, I would let my clients' words, feelings, and experiences guide our discussions as they developed.

Benji, one of the three clients in my group that evening, unknowingly chose the topic for our group process when, upon my asking him to share aloud what was on his mind, he begrudgingly responded with, "I don't want to feel this way!"

Benji was a young man with an affinity for ecstasy. He had danced through the last few years of his life in a haze of MDMA-fueled euphoria, masking his depression and constant inability to feel pleasure in life (or really feel anything at all) with three a.m. beach raves and heading an underground drug exchange. When those seven words left his mouth, I felt the energy in the room between the four of us shift.

The other two clients were Marcus and Emily. Marcus was a man in his fifties, haunted by a history of trauma, who sought relief from feeling through alcohol. Emily, an elderly woman, was grappling with decades of chronic pain, which led her to turn to heroin in a desperate attempt to silence the physical agony that constantly took over her mind.

We were all moved by Benji's vulnerable statement. We knew this phrase and what it meant for it to be said. When it comes to being human, not wanting to feel a certain way is the precursor to getting completely out of control.

I stood up, went to the whiteboard, grabbed a marker, and wrote in large capital letters, "I DON'T WANT TO FEEL THIS WAY!" We were going to talk about this for the next forty-five minutes, and they were on board. I listened to each of them, nodding and responding in empathy and understanding, as their stories unfolded. It made sense. Of course it did. We don't want to feel a stubbed toe—why would we want to feel depressed, traumatized, or chronically in pain?

The details they shared with me during our almost hour-long conversation aren't important for you to read. Why? Because they were shared in confidence, for one, and two, this book isn't about the specific experience of numbing feelings with substances. It's about you existing as a human being who feels. Who sometimes wants to and sometimes doesn't. Who may choose to numb how you feel, consciously or unconsciously, with substances, with alternative feelings, with distractions, with people, places, and things.

While the details *they* shared aren't crucial for your healing journey, what *I* shared during that group session is. I shared with Benji, Marcus, and Emily the concept of the somatic unconscious and how it lives within the body. And it impacted them so much that they've each separately reached out over the last ten years, reminding me of that night's group.

Remember, the **somatic unconscious** is made up of the *sensations* and *reactions* that occur in your body and brain without your conscious awareness or control—it's the term that encompasses how you stay alive without trying to (feeling, breathing, digesting). It's comprised of your somatic perceptions, physiological processes, nonverbal cues, and nervous system reactions.

SOMATIC UNCONSCIOUS: bodily reactions and sensations *that occur without your conscious awareness or control*

You likely understand that you have a body, that your body feels, and that it has reactions and sensations. I mean, it's a pretty hard thing to ignore, right? Wrong.

Have you ever noticed how the air you breathe into your nose is colder than the air you breathe out of it? Did you know you can always tap into that sensation?[2] Try it now. Place your attention on the sensation of air going into and then out of your nose. Feel the temperature difference. Cooler going in, warmer going out.

Now think about the next two birthdays you have coming up in your life. Whose birthdays are they? Is one of them yours? How are you feeling about these birthdays coming up? Do you need to get gifts? Will there be a party for one of them? For both?

While you were thinking about the answers to those questions, were you still actively feeling the temperature changes happening in your nose from your breathing? I'd bet on your answer being no. The thing is, that feeling, the nasal temperature change, was still there. It was still being felt by your somatic unconscious, relayed to your brain, yet not being actively experienced by your conscious mind. You didn't choose to *ignore* the sensation; you just moved your attention elsewhere. It's not that the air stopped changing temperature; it's that you stopped being consciously aware of it. You allowed the sensation to enter your consciousness when I asked you to, and then once you shifted your attention, your somatic unconscious took back over, monitoring it *for you*.

Your somatic unconscious is powerful. It takes care of so much. Think about how ridiculously exhausting it would be to have to actively, consciously monitor the temperature of air going into and out of your nose. Add on telling yourself, "Left foot, right foot, left foot, right foot," or "Mmm, I'm not feeling too hungry yet in this moment, and not in this moment, or this moment" on top of tracking your nasal airflow. We'd absolutely be a less capable species. There's no way we could have made the technological advances we have if our entire consciousness were spent on making sure our body was working correctly down to every subtle shift or change in sensation.

The work of the somatic unconscious is to track all the things going on inside and outside of your body, communicate what it realizes is happening with your brain, and help you stay safe, balanced, and healthy without you having to constantly think about how to do it on your own. It might not seem like the biggest deal that your somatic unconscious tracks the temperature of the air going into and out of your nose, but when you broaden the concept, you'll not only see how absolutely vital your somatic unconscious is but also how critical it is that you are aware of and work with it.

TRUTH TAKEAWAY: Feeling is part of being alive. Your body feels to help you, even though it sucks sometimes. Let yourself feel. You have to.

Drugs, like the ones my clients were using, can certainly dull, numb, or enhance your ability to be aware of your body and to feel or not to feel. It's the reason we've used drugs as a species for as long as we have—to shift our consciousness in some way. But there are, in my opinion, other, more subtly, or at times very overtly, dangerous things in your life that affect your ability to hear the messages your body is sending you and control your body in the ways you should. Things like society as a whole—from our employment structures (like needing multiple jobs to make ends meet without being able to meet your basic needs) to our human rights policies (or the lack thereof, when it comes to protecting entire communities of humans) to subjective "value"-based violence (where physical abuse is okay as long as it will "help them learn"). The lifestyles we lead. The pressures we face. The permissions we give or take away from ourselves and other people to *actually* feel, to *actually* listen to the messages our soma, our physical body,[3] our somatic unconscious, is trying to send us.

We all have ways that we ignore, muffle, judge, and work against our somatic unconscious—like when we hold our bladder because it's not break time yet at work or when we stay in an uncomfortable position in a chair because we don't want people to think we're rude for making a sound during a presentation. In these instances, we're telling our somatic unconscious we don't want to hear it and we don't want to see it. We're not interested in consciously receiving its messages. We don't want to be aware of how we need to use the restroom or stretch our bodies. It's not the time. And unless it's a dire situation, after a short period, we tend to be able to forget (read: push back into our unconscious) what our body truly needs.

Your somatic unconscious isn't only showing when *you* receive its messages and refuse them or when *you* should receive its messages but you don't, it's also showing when your body is sensing and reacting in ways that *others* can see but you can't. It shows when you haven't eaten all day due to a work deadline, and you blame your current bad mood on the impeding project and your asshole boss instead of your need for a snack. Next, you're thanking the colleague who passed you a granola bar in the hallway after saying, "You seem hangry" for helping you feel better.

Hangry: when you're angry because you're hungry. Yes, it's a real thing.[4]

Your somatic unconscious is showing when you think you're hiding how bored you are talking to a neighbor when in reality, it looks like an alien has sucked your brain right out of your skull, and you're dissociatively staring at them like they're a wall with white paint drying on it.

It shows when you're on stage and you aren't telling the audience you're nervous but they can see the sweat beads, notice your pacing increase, and hear the subtle stumbles your words are taking.

> **KNOW YOUR TERMS:** Dissociative: A state of your brain when it temporarily detaches from your immediate experiences, making you feel separated from your inner or outer environment.

Your somatic unconscious functions automatically, without your deliberate control or conscious decision-making. It responds to various stimuli, emotions, and situations, and we're usually not aware of its reactions until after the fact, if at all.

Your Inner Orchestra

Imagine your body as an orchestra, with every part from organs to cells playing its own special tune. Together, they create the complex (and essential) performance that is your body's functioning.

Just like a well-executed concert, when the systems in your body are in harmony, the result can be one of the most beautiful sounds you've ever heard—like a "Fuuuuck yes!" resulting from an orgasm. But what happens when the conductor starts ignoring complete sections of the orchestra or when someone or something distracts the conductor, moving their attention away from a certain system, causing it to fall out of tune or become dysregulated?

Before we answer that question, let's look at ten various systems your somatic unconscious tracks in, around, and for your body, i.e., the symphony sections of your bodily orchestra.

1. **When You're in Pain:** When your body is in pain, it communicates with your brain, telling it to assess and respond to potential threats or injuries. This is also known as nociception.[5]
2. **How Hot and Cold You Are:** Your body can feel sensations of

warmness or coldness, which give you information about the type of environment you're in and help your brain regulate your body temperature and respond accordingly. Also called thermoception.[6]

3. **When You Feel Touch and Pressure:** Different sensations of touch and pressure tell your brain how much physical contact you're receiving and information about the objects around you. Another name for this is mechanoreception.[7]

4. **Where Your Body Is Located:** Your brain and body communicate about your body's position in space, helping with balance, coordination, and movement. Also referred to as proprioception.[8]

5. **How Hungry or Thirsty You Are:** Body signals related to hunger and thirst guide your brain to ensure you give yourself essential nutrients and hydration.

6. **If Your Vitals Are Stable:** Your cardiovascular and respiratory systems constantly provide information about your heart rate, blood pressure, and oxygen levels.

7. **The Amount of Tension You Feel:** Feedback about muscle tension and relaxation helps your brain control your posture and manage stress.

8. **What You're Sensing:** Information from your five senses—sight, sound, taste, smell, and touch—shapes how you perceive the world around you.

9. **How Much Energy You Have or Need:** Your body's energy levels and feelings of sleepiness help your brain manage when you stay awake and when you need rest.

10. **If You Need to Use the Restroom:** When you need to urinate or defecate, your brain signals you to take action to keep yourself clean and healthy.

Pay attention to what are listed as the outcomes of these systems when they're acknowledged and working properly: the ability to respond to threats, help you balance, give yourself essential nutrients, manage your stress levels, maintain bodily hygiene, and more. So, what happens when you stop paying or refuse to pay conscious attention to, to be the conductor of, these systems? Well, the opposite happens.

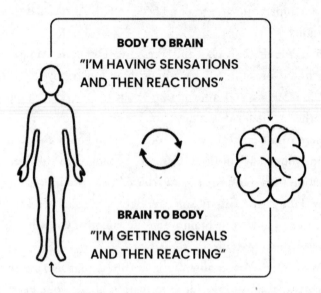

Your body finds ease in keeping you alive through a process called somatic sensory integration. **Somatic sensory integration** occurs when your brain receives, interprets, and responds to the messages sent by your somatic unconscious.[9] This interplay between your brain and body shapes your experiences, your emotions, and your behaviors.

When somatic integration is working well, you feel stable and in tune with yourself. But when you're upset by distress, distractions, trauma, or other issues, your inner harmony can turn into a mess, causing emotional overwhelm, physical pain, and a feeling of being out of touch with what's happening to you.

The relationship and communication between your body and brain occur on a spectrum. Some humans struggle to tune in to their bodies because they've become wired to focus only on the external. Some are completely detached, dissociated. On the other end, some people experience heightened sensitivity—where the body's soundtrack is turned on max volume, making it near impossible to stay grounded. I call the process of seeing where you land on this spectrum the **Internal Vibe Check.**

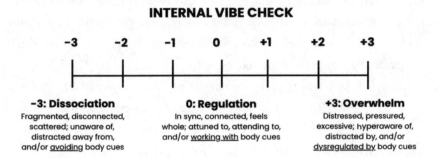

INTERNAL VIBE CHECK

| -3 | -2 | -1 | 0 | +1 | +2 | +3 |

−3: Dissociation
Fragmented, disconnected, scattered; unaware of, distracted away from, and/or <u>avoiding</u> body cues

0: Regulation
In sync, connected, feels whole; attuned to, attending to, and/or <u>working with</u> body cues

+3: Overwhelm
Distressed, pressured, excessive; hyperaware of, distracted by, and/or <u>dysregulated by</u> body cues

Under normal circumstances, you want to find yourself somewhere near the middle of this spectrum—where you're regulated, feel connected to your body, and are attuned to its needs. Your consciousness is listening to your somatic unconscious, and they're working together in harmony.

In some situations, individuals may have sensory processing disorders or difficulties that not only make it more challenging to integrate body sensations overall but also make it harder to regulate (and easier to dissociate or become overwhelmed) in circumstances others may not.

In other situations, it's most appropriate to find yourself dissociating or feeling overwhelmed—like if you're being physically harmed, dissociation will help you feel less pain, or if you're standing on the edge of a cliff, feeling overwhelmed by the wobbliness and increased heart rate makes sense.

> **MAKE IT SIMPLE:** You body's sensations, and your brain's reactions to them, vary, and they should. You don't want to be nonresponsive to life; you want to control your responses.

It's not about staying near zero; it's about being able to notice where you're at on the spectrum at any given time and moving closer to zero when it makes sense so you can be in control.

The spectrum within the Internal Vibe Check is similar to that of Dan Siegel's Window of Tolerance, a scale that helps people understand how they can stay within a range of emotional control where they're neither too overwhelmed nor too shut down to function well.[10] Dan's perspective is helpful when it comes to clinical populations and for those who have experienced notable shifts in their nervous system due to personally traumatic experiences.

And, fundamentally, every human being has a way they respond to their body's sensations, even if they've never had trauma. I say, "Get overwhelmed sometimes," "Activate dissociation when you need to." We have the ability to feel these ways for a reason.

Caring about how your body and brain interact with each other is fundamental, not reactionary. Knowing how and when you get overwhelmed and dissociative is important, as is giving yourself room to feel that way and know it's appropriate. The time to care about your somatic unconscious isn't just when you've experienced trauma, been diagnosed with a condition, or learned your attachment style; the time to care is always, from the moment you were born a human on this planet.

> **TRUTH TAKEAWAY:** It's not always about what happened to you; sometimes it's just about who you are. Don't judge every way your body and brain react as negative or problematic or trauma-related. It's not.

People think the human brain developed to help the body react to the world around it, explicitly. It didn't.

Two scenarios:

1. You hear someone scream, look to your right, and there's a car about to hit you.
   Your cognitive unconscious: Quick, jump out of the way!
   Your somatic unconscious: Okay!
   Your consciousness: *Thank goodness!*
2. You're watching a movie, someone screams, the main character looks to their right, and, suddenly, there's a car about to hit them.
   Your cognitive unconscious: Quick, jump out of the way!
   Your somatic unconscious: Okay!

>Your consciousness: . . . *You were fine. You were in a comfy*
>*theater, logically and rationally safe from getting hit by any vehicles,*
>*and you still jumped.*

Similar reactions, but only one was accurate and actually needed. The point: Your brain did not evolve to react to your world; it evolved as a prediction machine to save your life through the regulation and use of your body—and sometimes those predictions are wrong.

Your brain keeps your body alive not by perceiving the world around you correctly and in real time, but by regulating your body in anticipation of your future needs, preparing to meet them *before* they arise—a process known as allostasis.

You've probably heard of homeostasis—your body's natural tendency to maintain stability or equilibrium in its internal environment. It regulates things like your body temperature, blood pressure, and glucose levels. It's where your body likes to be at baseline.

Allostasis, on the other hand, is your body's unconscious ability to physiologically *adapt* to stressors or challenges—like when it uses your fight-flight-freeze response to attack, run, or hide in a dangerous situation—and then return to baseline.[11] And interoception—awareness of your body sensations and signals[12] (i.e., *conscious* somatic sensory integration)—is a direct result of this ability. First, be aware. Then, be in control.

> **MAKE IT SIMPLE:** Because your body reacts to what happens
> in- and outside of it (allostasis), you can use interoception
> (being conscious of your body) to stay balanced and in control
> (homeostasis).

When completing an Internal Vibe Check, you're engaging in interoception, and there are two ways to do it. The first is to consider the relationship with your body and what it's like when you're at interoceptive baseline and homeostatic balance—meaning when you're not experiencing anything scary or exciting, for example, that throws you off and makes you feel or react in a way atypical to how you normally do.

I want you to explore your overall level of somatic sensory integration.

At any given (non-stressful or emotional) moment, how are you relating to and regulating your body? How often are you checking in with it, and what is the reaction when you do so? Do you *like* feeling the vibe of your own existence? Why or why not?

Then, think about all the messages your body sends your brain that help keep you alive, like how fast your heart is beating and how much pressure is on your body. Let's use the examples of when you're in pain and how hungry and thirsty you are.

When something seemingly painful is happening to your body, are you able to regulate your response? Do the pain signals overwhelm you, or is it actually hard to feel them?

With hunger and thirst, do you often find yourself only becoming conscious of these needs when they reach a level of sickness? Do you actively ignore these specific somatic messages, or do they take you over?

Explore, consciously, your somatic unconscious. Shine your flashlight beam on that part of your warehouse. Explore the body of the car. Feel that part of the elephant.

Then, choose your baseline vibe.

Baseline Internal Vibe Check: Where do you land on the scale *most* days, in *most* situations, with *most* sensations?

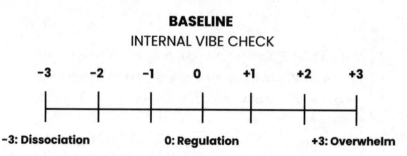

BASELINE
INTERNAL VIBE CHECK

| -3 | -2 | -1 | 0 | +1 | +2 | +3 |

-3: Dissociation   **0: Regulation**   **+3: Overwhelm**

The second way to complete your Internal Vibe Check involves when you want to gauge how your somatic unconscious is showing (and altering your perception of what's happening) during a specific situation. Maybe you find yourself in a state of overwhelm or dissociation at baseline, or perhaps you find yourself entering into a state of dissociation or overwhelm, and are wanting to move into self-regulation mode. This could be any type of situation, from feeling anxious when trying to make a tough decision to experiencing unexpected anger to the onset of a panic attack.

Situational Internal Vibe Check: Where are you on the scale *right now*, in *this* situation, with *these* sensations?

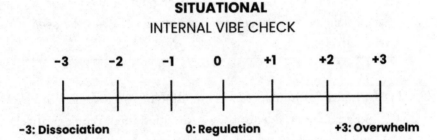

SITUATIONAL
INTERNAL VIBE CHECK

-3   -2   -1   0   +1   +2   +3

-3: Dissociation   0: Regulation   +3: Overwhelm

The goal in knowing both of these numbers (your baseline and situational vibe) is to simply know yourself enough to control yourself. If you aren't happy with where you find yourself at baseline or in any given situation, make a note to work on this during your journey through the 12 Steps of Consciousness.

The Internal Vibe Check isn't just something that can be used for your solo benefit. It can also be used in relationships of all kinds—with friends, family, romantic partners, and colleagues. My husband and I have used this checking system for over a year now, and it's been a game changer.

When shit hits the fan, we've learned that he tends to—starting from his self-reported baseline of 0 (Mr. Regulated over there)—land somewhere between +1 (mostly attuned, slightly overwhelmed) and +1.5 (at risk of becoming moderately distressed and dysregulated—usually when I move from *my* baseline and make things worse).

At baseline, you can find me at -1.5 (moderately dissociated and ignoring my bodily cues). When things go awry, I'm, at worst, quick to slide to +2.5 (moderately or severely overwhelmed), and at best, hover around -1 or +1 (when using successful conscious control at work and/or when my children are involved).* We use the communication of our internal vibes to share what our somatic unconscious is doing, what's controlling us, and what we're trying to control ourselves. This leads to us understanding each other more, and respecting and supporting the current state each of our bodies and brains are in.

> **TRUTH TAKEAWAY:** Sharing the messages that your body sends your brain with your partner is like teaching them the language of your stability. You show them how to see what can't be seen on the outside.

In 2019, at the International Convention of Psychological Science (ICPS) in Paris, the president of the Association for Psychological Science, Lisa Feldman Barrett, said, "Your body is part of your mind, not in some gauzy mystical way, but in a very real biological way. This means there is a piece of your body in every concept that you make, even in states that we think of as cold cognition."[13]

What she's saying is that you don't have thoughts or behaviors that aren't, in some way, influenced by how your body feels and that there's a piece of your body in every concept you form, even in cognitive processes you think of as rational or analytical. She's saying the somatic unconscious exists, is important, and is controlling you. Even if you don't want to accept that as fact, it still is.

You are the conscious conductor of your inner orchestra. You are the *only* person who can hear the music, feel the sensations, and control what happens next.

It's Not All in Your Head (or Inside Your Body)

One obvious downside to your somatic unconscious: Others can see it, even when you can't (or won't).

---

* I am as consciously controlled as I can be around my children. It's my number one goal as a parent, alongside teaching them how to do the same.

In the group that day in late 2015, I knew how Emily, the older woman using heroin to numb her chronic pain, was feeling before she said a word. I could see it even though she couldn't. When Benji said, "I don't want to feel this way," Emily initially responded verbally with silence but, at the same time, at least from my perspective, *screamed* with her body. She shifted her seat position, took off her jacket, rolled her eyes, started taking deep, sigh-like breaths, and then, after all of that, she finally replied with, "At least you feel numbness and not pain!"

I didn't know exactly what she was going to say, but by the way her body was responding, it was easy to cut my mental list down to something unsettled, heavy, and unwanted.

It can be beneficial when your somatic unconscious shows in a therapeutic setting. It gives you the opportunity to show more of yourself to those who are trying to help you gain control. Emily and I, in group, along with Benji and Marcus, processed how her body responded to what Benji said *before* she became consciously aware of her own feelings. This led her to the realization that her body had her back—literally and *figuratively*—a perspective she hadn't been able to take since the onset of her chronic physical illness six years prior.

Just as Emily didn't decide how her somatic unconscious showed in that moment, there will be moments you can't, either. Honestly, it will probably be most of your moments. Even, at times, the big ones.

A year before I ran that group, an incident unfolded at the 2014 Consumer Electronics Show (CES) that showcases how even the most seasoned professionals can have their somatic unconscious show, putting them in unexpected and uncomfortable situations.

Michael Bay is an American filmmaker and director, whose name is synonymous with high-octane action and explosive spectacles. He's best known for creating scenes that include quick edits and polished visuals—think *Pearl Harbor* or *Transformers*. But this day, things were more explosive and quick than they were polished.

The CES is an event where technology giants present their latest innovations. On this particular day, Michael was invited to speak about his experiences with high-definition television and filmmaking. However, what was supposed to be a routine appearance took an unexpected turn.

His teleprompter stopped working. The one that had his script on it. The audience couldn't see it working or not working. Only Michael could. But what the audience *could* see was likely everything I'd assume he wished they couldn't.

As soon as the teleprompter malfunctioned, Michael's discomfort was immediately visible. He appeared tense and uncertain, which was evident in his posture and facial expressions.

He was pacing back and forth on the stage, leading many to think he was nervous or lacked confidence in himself or his presentation. At times, he raised his arms in a gesture of frustration. He looked helpless, and it looked like he felt that way, too.

The worst display of his somatic unconscious was when it caused him to look in the complete opposite direction of the audience, toward the back of the stage, multiple times. From the audience's point of view, something was clearly wrong.

The experience seemed to become too much for Michael, and although it appeared he attempted to consciously glance at some notes he had on the podium, his uncontrolled, non-curated somatic unconscious had gotten the best of him. He gave up, said, "I'm sorry," and abruptly left the stage.*

His hasty departure was a clear indicator that something had gone terribly wrong, but there was more to the story than just a technological glitch. More parts to consider, more dark corners of the warehouse to explore.

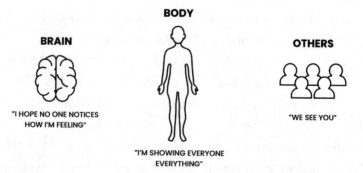

BODY

BRAIN

OTHERS

"I HOPE NO ONE NOTICES
HOW I'M FEELING"

"WE SEE YOU"

"I'M SHOWING EVERYONE
EVERYTHING"

---

* Michael, I've been here. No judgment. We're all human. Thanks for your great movies.

Nonverbal communication encompasses the various ways we convey information and emotions without using words.[14] It is a vital part of human interaction, often conveying more than just talking could by itself. Michael's struggle on the CES stage offers a prime example of unconscious nonverbal cues taking center stage in a high-stress situation.

Here's a list of various types of unconscious nonverbal communication you're likely using:

1. **Facial Expressions:** These can and will range. Your face can either be incredibly expressive and convey a wide range of emotions, from joy and excitement to frustration and embarrassment, or you can have a case of resting bitch face—where, when relaxing all your facial muscles, you look consistently pissed. (This is me, but you usually can't tell unless I'm stuck in dissociation mode at a -2.)

   Pay attention to the face you're making at any given time. It can sometimes say more than your words do.

2. **Overall Body Language:** Body language encompasses posture, gestures, and movements. For example, Emily's physical readjustment on the couch in the group, the removal of her jacket, and the rolling of her eyes were all body language manifestations of her somatic unconscious revealing her upset.[15]

   You can consciously use your body to your advantage, or it can take advantage of you, gaining its own comfort while making public your private emotions.

3. **Eye Contact:** The way you use eye contact can communicate interest, engagement, or discomfort. In Michael's case, I doubt he was consciously telling himself, "Look away from the audience. You don't see them, they don't see you." This was an important moment for him, and avoidance of eye contact indicated his potential unease with his audience.

   Keep in mind eye contact holds different levels of comfort for different types of people.

4. **Tone of Voice:** Although not strictly nonverbal, tone of voice is also not always in our conscious control. Changes in tone can

convey emotions like anger, nervousness, or confidence. Think about a time when you were pissed but didn't want to show it. Sometimes it gets to the point where we're literally talking through our teeth to feel in control of our voice.

This is a good one to pay attention to when in a conversation to sense if you or any of the other people are starting to shift toward an argument without knowing it yet.

5. **Proximity:** How close or far you stand from someone can convey comfort or discomfort. Have you ever experienced stepping back, away from someone or something, without consciously telling yourself to? Or what about finding yourself sitting two inches closer to the person you're crushing on an hour into the movie you're watching, even though you don't recall ever deciding to make the night cozier?

We have unconscious sensors for proximity in our body and brain. It's part of why we can *sense* when someone is behind us or looking at us. Your somatic unconscious knows they're there, but conscious you hasn't actually looked yet—it's, shall we say, your . . . Spidey-sense (if you use it wisely).[16]

Nonverbal behaviors can be conscious or unconscious. Communication is deeply intertwined with your mental and emotional state. Your mental health can affect nonverbal communication not only in high-pressure situations like Michael's or highly emotional situations like group therapy but also in your everyday interactions.

For individuals dealing with conditions like anxiety or depression, our nonverbal cues may subtly reveal our emotional states, impacting how others perceive and respond to us, especially when we aren't (or can't) verbally communicating what's going on inside. However, keep in mind that we, individually, will assume what someone else's nonverbals mean. And we could be wrong. We often are.

Understanding the significance of nonverbal communication is valuable for both your personal and professional growth. To help you explore yours, here's an exercise that could fuck with your head in an irreversible way, change your life in a good way, or both (hopefully both). It's called Third-Person Mirror.

Third-Person Mirror: Have someone record you for an entire day, or record yourself if you think you'd act more natural. Record as much of your day as possible, excluding moments of privacy or confidentiality—like work calls or using the restroom.*

Then, play back the recording. You don't need to do this in real-time speed; it could be hours of footage. You can speed it up and look for patterns. Pay attention to what you thought you were thinking and doing in certain moments and if it looks like you may have actually been doing or feeling something different.

THIRD PERSON MIRROR EXERCISE

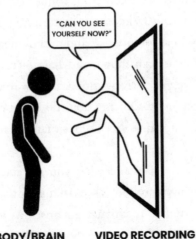

BODY/BRAIN   **VIDEO RECORDING**

Upon reflection, ask yourself:

What do your nonverbal behaviors reveal about you?

Though fair warning before you begin: There's a reason I said it could fuck with your head. This is one of the interventions my husband used on me during the ultimatum phase of my life and our relationship.

---

* Then again, you *could* film your facial expressions in the restroom; it'd be a curious move, but you may learn a lot . . .

He recorded me in a deep blackout—when a person drinks so much alcohol they don't remember what happened. I had almost no ability to consciously control my nonverbal responses, let alone the verbal ones.

Alcohol shuts down your prefrontal cortex—a part of your brain that contributes to higher-order cognitive functions, like decision-making, planning, and, as far as we know today, *consciousness*. If the prefrontal cortex is shut down or impaired, it can lead to difficulty making rational decisions, controlling impulses, and maintaining a coherent sense of self-awareness.

In short: My video was a damn disaster. It was by far the most embarrassing thing I had ever watched of myself in my life. It's part of why I took the ultimatum so seriously.

Other things shown to shut down or impair the functioning of the prefrontal cortex (i.e., make conscious control more difficult), other than alcohol, include stress, fatigue, traumatic brain injuries, dehydration, hunger, anger, other substance use, and overall mental illness. The Third-Person Mirror exercise can show you what you're like in many different states of being, from excessively intoxicated to mildly stressed or falling in love. Don't sleep on it. Oh, and don't do it to a partner or friend without their permission. Mine was a dire situation, and my husband did it as a last resort.

If you do this exercise, and what you see alarms you, know you're not alone. Exploring your body's sensations, watching yourself from the outside, and meeting your somatic unconscious is trippy, can be scary, and also can be wildly illuminating. So, like I said, don't sleep on it, but try to make sure it doesn't become a living nightmare.

The Bridge of Seduction

Speaking of living nightmares, let's talk about my parents.*

Just kidding, we're not going to talk about them like that. They aren't nightmares—but they are alive!

---

* I love my parents, and it hasn't been the easiest to have them as parents or for them to have me as a child because I . . . was and am a "hard" daughter, to say the least.

Although my parents and I have had difficulties throughout our thirty-plus years together, we've also managed to have some really great experiences. They met during their high school years, had me shortly after, never married, haven't been together my entire life, and I've somehow ended up in the exact same location with each of them separately, during different periods of my life.

The location? The Capilano Suspension Bridge Park in North Vancouver, Canada.

The main attraction of this park is in its name—the Capilano Suspension Bridge. Since 1889, this bridge, spanning 450 feet long and wobbling 230 feet above the ground, has been daring people to cross it.

The thought of crossing this bridge intrigued my father when I visited the park with him in 2007—I, on the other hand, a sixteen-year-old who had never done anything remotely physical regarding heights, was terrified. My father's always been the type of person who knows and understands how to use his body, whether that be strength, movement, etc., to his advantage. To him, the bridge was a fun yet scary challenge. To me, it was a challenge to even consider that I might survive if I stepped foot on it. While the experience of me crossing was tense and slow, I eventually made it to the other side. It was easy enough that I was eventually convinced to do it again.

For my mother, the bridge was, in fact, her living nightmare. My mother has always had a fear of heights. I visited the bridge with her in 2017, ten years after visiting with my father. I had a conscious memory of my past experience, so this time around, I was interested in shaking things up—pun intended—as my mother was crossing the bridge. I took pleasure in rocking it a bit behind her and telling her to "look out" and "hold on." It wasn't very nice, and it was meant to be—and ended up being—innocuous and playful in the end. It took her three times as long to cross as it did my father. However, this means nothing other than the fact that different people have different experiences on this bridge and for different reasons.

This bridge is scary. It's long, tall, and in the middle of a forest. It's not meant to just be a beautiful experience. It's meant to make you have, at minimum, an exhilarating somatic experience. The bridge activates you and changes you, both in the moment and, at times, indefinitely. How?

When it comes to the human condition, your emotions, thoughts, and behaviors are not isolated islands—they aren't separated. They are interconnected, influenced by the ever-present dialogue between your body, brain, and mind.

Let's journey through the famous study by Dutton and Aron,[17] a study that took place on the Capilano Suspension Bridge in 1974, which shows how misinterpreting the sensations in your body can affect how attractive you find other people. For those of you currently seeking a partner, pay attention.

To understand the study's context, picture this: a rickety suspension bridge swaying high above a terrifying cliff. A group of male participants is told to sightsee at the park and cross the bridge. After crossing the bridge, a good-looking woman (a researcher who's secretly part of the study) approaches the participants, they chat, and she asks them to write a short story about an ambiguous picture she shows them. She hands them her number afterward, offering the opportunity to call her regarding any questions about her "project." That's half the study.

During the other half, a different group of men undergoes the same experience with the woman who's in on the study—except they aren't 230 feet in the air. There's a less intimidating, more stable bridge these guys walk across before meeting the woman.

Now, here's where it gets intriguing. After both bridge encounters, each group's stories were assessed along with tracking which men ended up calling the phone number provided by the attractive woman. The results were eye-opening. Men who crossed the suspension bridge generally presented more sexualized stories, along with 50 percent of these men giving the woman researcher a call, compared to about 13 percent of those who crossed the shorter one, who also had less sexualized stories.

But why would a taller, scarier bridge make the men call the woman more often, and think more sexually during their storytelling?

Dutton and Aron suggest that the thrill of crossing the shaky bridge caused physical signs of arousal like a faster heartbeat and sweating, which the men mistook for attraction to the woman, not realizing it was actually anxiety from the bridge.

> **MAKE IT SIMPLE:** Your brain may not correctly interpret what your body is trying to say. Be mindful of the stories you attach to how your body feels.

The misattribution of arousal led them to perceive the woman as more attractive than they might have under different circumstances.* Misattribution of arousal isn't just a psychological phenomenon confined to laboratory experiments; it frequently plays out in our daily lives, sometimes with amusing or unexpected results.

Most people believe that when we experience emotions, it's a simple cause-and-effect process. Something happens, and then we feel a corresponding emotion. For example, if something irritating occurs, we get angry, or if something delightful happens, we feel happy.

However, our bodies don't always follow this logical path. Instead of feeling distinct emotions like anger or happiness, most of the time, we experience something more basic: arousal. And then, we give it another, more specific name based on what's going on around us at the time. While the term "arousal" is often associated with sex, it essentially refers to heightened physiological responses such as increased blood pressure, heart rate, and sensory alertness. When our bodies get aroused, it's not always immediately clear what caused it; and (this is a big point to make) your body can get aroused even when your mind isn't at all.

Here's some manipulative dating advice: The next time you want to unconsciously convince your date that you're "the one," choose an activity for the two of you that's meant to generally arouse your bodies—roller coasters, scary movies, escape rooms. If your date hasn't

---

* Maybe I should try this experiment on my parents and see if I can get them to like each other again . . . A girl can dream.

read this book, they just may fall in love with you even if you're not their type.*

To prove I'm joking, here's some advice that's helpful (because that's always more ethical coming from a therapist): If you're the one being asked on a date, and you're unsure of whether you really like the person asking you out, don't be fooled—settle for a coffee date (decaf; caffeine will get you aroused)—or something else less activating; and if you want to go on the more action-packed date, remember that your somatic unconscious shows, look for it, and remind yourself that *conscious you* is going to decide if you like them, not your body.

TRUTH TAKEAWAY: People who know more about how your body and brain work than you do may be using that knowledge to manipulate you. Keep learning about yourself to maintain control.

Dutton and Aron's findings from the Capilano Bridge study were interpreted using the two-factor theory of emotion,[18] which suggests that there are two factors that play a role in our emotional experiences at humans.

Emotion Factor 1: Physiological arousal: bodily reactions and sensations

Emotion Factor 2: Cognitive interpretation: mental perceptions and information processing

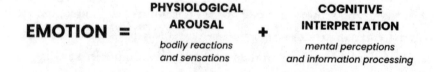

EMOTION = **PHYSIOLOGICAL AROUSAL** + **COGNITIVE INTERPRETATION**
bodily reactions and sensations   *mental perceptions and information processing*

While we're going to discuss your cognitive unconscious and how it affects your interpretation of the world in the next chapter, let's look at one more study to help you understand how your body and brain create your perceptions.

---

* Obviously, I mean this jokingly. Don't manipulate people. Use your superpowers for good, not evil.

The two-factor theory of emotion was developed by Stanley Schachter and Jerome Singer in the early 1960s. They conducted a similar experiment in which they injected their participants with a hormone (epinephrine) that caused them to experience arousal—increased heart rate and trembling hands. Then, they stuck these people next to someone else who was secretly a part of the study. This person was instructed to act either happy or angry. At the end of the experiment, when asked how they were feeling, the participants near the person acting happy reported feeling happy, while those next to the person acting angry reported feeling angry. Same physiological responses, totally opposite somatic unconscious interpretations—their conscious brains experienced entirely different emotions.

The key finding was that the participants' emotional reactions depended on the situation and context. If the people you surround yourself with can influence how you perceive your own body's messages that much, it kind of makes you want to review everyone you hang out with and make sure they aren't poisoning your mind, doesn't it? (And don't even get me started on your social media following.)

> **KNOW YOUR TERMS:** Situation and context: The specific conditions, circumstances, and background that create or influence an event or action.

A final metaphor: Imagine you're asked to make a cake for a neighbor's family gathering. All you're told about the attendees of the gathering is that they're going to be experiencing racing hearts, possible sweating, shallow or deep breathing, and there will probably be tears. According to this two-factor theory of emotion, you'll need to know more about the context of these people's experiences before you can actually make the cake. Is it a wedding, and these physiological responses are of a joyous, slightly apprehensive form? Or is it a funeral, and a three-tier, red velvet wedding cake with confetti that pops out would be the last thing the family wants?

Emotions aren't just about how your body feels or what's in your somatic unconscious; they also depend on what's happening around you and how your brain is making sense of everything. If you'd ask questions to make sure this family got the type of cake they needed, you should probably start asking yourself questions, too.

Instead of allowing your somatic unconscious to hand you a predetermined assumption of what your feelings are and what they're saying you need or want, try, like I did that night in the group with Benji, Marcus, and Emily, "working with what's in the room," except for you, the room is your body, and your clients are your internal systems.

Let both your somatic sensations *and* your cognitive interpretations guide your understanding of reality. But be wary—your cognition is not always in your control, either, as you'll soon learn in the next chapter.

CHAPTER 3 SUMMARY

- You don't always like the way you feel, and that's fine. It's human.
- Your somatic unconscious keeps you alive. It tracks everything from pain to energy levels and whether you're hungry or not.
- Your body has a mind (and a voice) of its own. Listen to it.
- Every thought and behavior you have is influenced by your body.
- You say a lot more than just the words that come out of your mouth.

4

You Are Biased

The Cognitive Unconscious

Do you perceive the world as it is—*objectively*?

The hard truth: not really.

Here's a simple explanation for how you, a human with a brain, construct reality: Your body sends signals to your brain, and then, in combination with signals coming from your environment, your brain tries to make sense of it all—its outcome is your reality.

You see reality through a subjective lens made up of how *you* feel, what *you* interpret, and the experiences *you* have.

Your body has eyes; your brain doesn't. Your body feels things; your brain doesn't. Your body moves; your brain doesn't. Your brain only experiences the electrochemical changes that are taking place within it—the outcome of said sensory signals—*not* the sensations themselves. Your brain is constantly guessing what's happening.

If your brain only had the information from the signals that were *currently* happening to make its guesses, it wouldn't make the best ones. The good thing is that your brain has other pieces of information it can use. One vital piece is that of *past* experiences and the information they've provided you.

But there's a major issue, and it's one that doesn't just make it hard for *you* to determine what's happening in your *own* reality, but one that's also made it hard for researchers to study other people's reality (even when looking at actual brain scans). They refer to this challenge as the reverse inference problem—a problem James is going to demonstrate for us.

James is an American neuroscientist currently working at the University of California, Irvine (UCI), just twenty minutes away from where I live.

One day, James was sitting at his desk sifting through brain scans. The brain scans were of all different types of people: people who presented with depression, some with schizophrenia, some who were "normal," and some . . . who were murderers. He was looking for specific parts of the brain that seemed linked to psychopathic behaviors.

Meanwhile, there was another stack of brain scans on his desk—his own and his family members. He had gathered these more personal scans for a separate study he was conducting on Alzheimer's markers, not psychopathy.

Upon reviewing all of his family's brain scans, toward the bottom of the pile he came across a clearly "abnormal" scan—one that showed reduced activity in areas of the frontal and temporal lobes (parts of the brain linked to self-control and empathy). This brain scan looked like the brain of a psychopath, though it shouldn't have—it was from the Alzheimer's pile.

Although the scans were supposed to be anonymous and confidential, because he knew this scan was from his family pile, he decided to look at whose it was.

He was shocked: It was his.

His first thought was that he'd misread the scan. "I've never killed anybody, or [sexually assaulted] anyone."[1] So, to him, these areas of the brain showing reduced activity (the frontal and temporal lobes) must *not* have been linked to psychopathy. But he wanted to be sure, so he decided to dig deeper. And it got worse.

First, he tested his genes. He found that he has the MAO-A gene, a gene linked to aggression and violence, among other genetic results. Then, he researched his family and discovered he is related to multiple high-profile murderers. Finally, he accepted that he does behave in ways many psychopaths are known to, like manipulating others. All of these findings led him to decide that he is a psychopath. Not a normal psychopath, but rather a "pro-social psychopath"—someone with the genetic makeup of a "born" psychopath but who was given love instead of abuse or neglect as a child.[2] Someone who can't feel true empathy but behaves in socially acceptable ways.[3]

All to say, James made a *reverse inference*—he assumed things about himself based on a brain scan. And intense, life-altering assumptions at that! However, the brain scan James used to come to this conclusion wasn't one that showed his brain activating during specific empathy tests, so it wasn't actually testing his ability to be empathetic or not[4] . . . Basically, the conclusion was a huge jump and the brain scan lacked significant evidence toward his point. He's not a true psychopath. He admits he's not. Yet he holds true that he "could have been."

> **MAKE IT SIMPLE:** You see the world through your own lens. Your brain takes your emotions, mixes them with your thoughts and your past, and spits out reality, but only *your* reality. We each have our own.

Does James's conclusion that he's a psychopath scare you? It scared James—so much so that now he consciously observes his behaviors to make sure he's acting in line with his values.[5] It doesn't scare me, even though he lives so close to me. And it doesn't scare Craig, a professor and researcher of neuroscience and behavior at UCI, who has an office across from James. Craig makes a great point when discussing this whole debacle: "What would happen if someone close to [James] were found dead under suspicious circumstances?"[6]

Would we decide he was guilty simply based on his brain scan and all the suggestive (and perceivably damning) "evidence" of him being a psychopath?

James believes it.

Or would we ensure, to the best of our abilities, that we were correct in our assumptions, judgments, and perceptions before convicting him of a specific, psychopathic crime?

These are not only problems we face in the courtroom; these are problems we face when using our own brains every day. We not only have difficulty figuring out what specific brain scans really mean, but we also have difficulty understanding what our brain is specifically scanning when it comes our interpretation of our experiences.

Our cognition—the mental process of acquiring, analyzing, and using information for various mental activities—allows us to perceive, sense, and process our inner and outer worlds. As it does this, as our brain undergoes its cognitive processes, it creates our reality. And, unless you're actively telling it what to do or at least watching the inferences it's making, it's doing it all unconsciously and out of your control.

A benefit of James being a neuroscientist is that he didn't stop at his brain scan before reaching his outcome. I'm not going to decide whether or not James could or could not have been a psychopath. I simply do not care. What I do care about, though, is that he, at least, went through a series of additional tests and inquiries before coming to his decided conclusion—that he's a "could-have-been" psychopath. Most of us don't do that before we make decisions, judge others, assume truths—that is, pause to rethink and gather more information—and we should.

Are you *sure* you want to vote that person into office, or have you just been persuaded by the constant availability of their campaign slogans plastered all over town?

Do you *really* need the latest iPhone to be your most productive self, or are you just succumbing to the allure of the familiar pattern of fall releases and talking about the updates with your friends (who also immediately made the purchase)?

Is that person *actually* a threat to you, or are you stereotyping them using only information that's been fed to you by those who want you to think that they are?

It's not likely that you're reading this book because you're trying to determine if you're a psychopath using your own brain scans. (Maybe, though. The book's title would lead it to not be an awful choice if you were.) It *is* likely that you're trying to determine, well, how you make determinations—how you choose what you think, how you judge people, and what you do or do not do. These are great questions to have.

The short answer to how you make decisions? You usually don't. Your cognitive unconscious does and it does it almost entirely on its own.

Your cognitive unconscious is made up of the *mental perceptions* and *information processing* that occur in your brain without your conscious awareness or control. Going back to the car metaphor from Chapter One, in the last chapter on the somatic unconscious, we explored the body of the car, including the physical engine. In this chapter, we're looking at how the engine, your brain, functions *systematically*—we're looking at its software and how it's programmed to work when on autopilot. How does it know which roads (which decisions) are the fastest, most efficient, and perceivably most desired, and why?

Your cognitive unconscious is, in itself, biased and selfish. It relies on deep-seated information and decision-making processes that are shaped by your past experiences, and its primary goal is to ensure the survival of your body and brain using the smallest amount of energy necessary.

When you think about your cognitive unconscious metaphorically, think about it using the principle of *the drunkard's search*.[7]

The drunkard is a man who was searching for something under a streetlight. When a police officer asked the man what he was looking for, he said his keys, and they both started looking together. After a few minutes, the policeman asked if the man was sure this was where he lost his keys. The man said, "No, I lost them in the park." When the officer asked the man why he wasn't searching there, he replied, "Because this is where the light is."[8]

The principle is this: Unconscious people tend to only look for something where it's easiest to look. And drunk or not, you're always 95 percent unconscious.

TRUTH TAKEAWAY: Your brain is stingy with its energy and indifferent when it comes to the truth. Don't rely heavily on what it can do on its own.

Quick!

Answer this question:

A bat and a ball cost $1.10 in total. The bat costs $1 more than the ball. How much does the ball cost?[9]

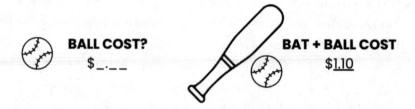

BALL COST?
$ _ . _ _

BAT + BALL COST
$1.10

The usual immediate answer is "10 cents." Which is a wrong but simpler conclusion to arrive at quickly: $1.10 can easily be cut down in the mind to $1.00 and 10 cents, and a 10-cent ball sounds reasonable in comparison to a $1 bat.[10]

Nonetheless, when you slow down and do the math, you're able to come to a more accurate answer (which is that the ball costs $0.05).*

Your cognitive unconscious is remarkable. It calculates the potential consequences of every action and thought in your day—such as the exact sequence of steps needed to tie your shoelaces and what happens when you throw a basketball at a certain time in a certain way to make a specific type of shot—at what seems like the speed of light. (In reality, we think much, much more slowly than that—around 270 miles per hour.)

Sure, it can be wrong sometimes. And other times, more curiously, it can convince you that you would've or could've become a psychopath in another lifetime. Regardless, as I've said, your unconscious is not a bad thing. Without it, we'd be overwhelmed, unable to function efficiently in a complex world.

Behind the scenes, your cognitive unconscious is busy picking up cues, weighing dangers, and smoothing over social situations. It's the source of your gut feelings, snap judgments, and fast choices. This inner software of yours makes life's complex navigation seem easy, as though

---

* The ball costs $0.05 and the bat costs $1.05. This makes the bat cost $1 more than the ball.

autopilot is the perfect guide, but it's not. Tuning into and consciously curating this part of you will help you make better decisions, avoid cognitive biases, and enhance your understanding of both yourself and the world around you.

Don't be caught acting drunk; take control of where you look for the truth. Don't be limited by your cognitive unconscious acting like a streetlight, limiting your vision to its own shallow perspective.

Fuck, Marry, Kill: Charlie, Nina, or Max?

What do a psychological social cognition theory and a popular teenage schoolyard game* have in common?

Nothing, but this section is going to include both.

| FUCK | MARRY | KILL |

First, the name of the game is "Fuck, Marry, Kill."[11] I'm going to describe three people to you, and after I do, you have to decide which of each of these individuals you would either fuck, marry, or kill. You can only pick one person for each category. Here we go.

Person #1: Charlie.

Charlie is a cognitive minimalist. He prefers shortcuts and quick thinking. He's been through enough in life to understand it *all* like the back of his hand. "All of what?" you might ask. Well, of everything. Charlie is an ego-inflated know-it-all (who, in fact, doesn't know it all). While he makes quick decisions, he doesn't remember the details of almost anything, can be super biased at times, and will act like he knows what he's talking about when he doesn't.

---

* Do I think this is the best "teenage schoolyard game"? No. Did I play it as a teen? Yes. Would I recommend it to or for a teen? No. Is it the *worst* game? It depends. Probably not.

Person #2: Nina.

Meet Nina, the meticulous thinker. She treats every situation (and I mean *every* situation) like a science experiment. She can't make a decision without knowing all the data, every potential perspective, and knowing all possible outcomes. She's pretty thorough and accurate, but she suffers from analysis paralysis and often struggles to actually make decisions fast enough.

And Person #3: Max.

Max is a versatile processor. He switches back and forth between quick thinking and in-depth analysis based on the demands of the situation. He's balanced, efficient, often accurate, and adaptive. This makes him an effective problem solver who knows when to trust what his intuition shows him and when to look inward and see what's going on.

Have your answers? Good.

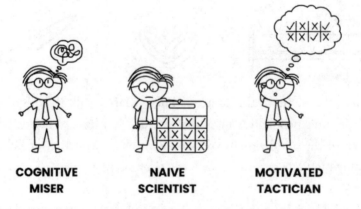

COGNITIVE   NAIVE   MOTIVATED
MISER   SCIENTIST   TACTICIAN

The game is "Fuck, Marry, Kill," and the theory is called attribution theory.

Attribution theory was developed in 1958 by Fritz Heider, who believed that people are motivated by two primary needs: the need to form a coherent view of the world and the need to be in control of their environment. Fritz believed that humans want and need consistency, stability, control, and the ability to accurately predict. In order to meet these needs, we make attributions[12]—judgments about whether the causes of what we're experiencing are internal or external (like your locus of control), stable or unstable, and controllable or uncontrollable, and so on. These attributions can be conscious or unconscious. He called the action of *consciously* fulfilling these cognitive needs with slow, active, and logical attributions being a "naive scientist."

Nina is a naive scientist. If I were you, I'd fuck Nina. It might take a while for her to get the hang of what's really going on, but she's likely to figure it out.

When we make attributions unconsciously, quickly, simply, using only past information and allowing for assumptions, we're giving our cognitive unconscious permission to make our decisions, judgments, and perceptions for us. We're acting like Charlie.

Charlie is a "cognitive miser."[13] We should absolutely kill Charlie. If anything, Charlie is one of those people who thought they were attracted to you because they misattributed their arousal not toward the tall bridge they were standing on but onto you, and they wouldn't even call you back after the first date.

There's only one person and one choice left: Marry Max. Marrying Max would be a really good idea, and not just by the process of elimination.

Max represents what's called a "motivated tactician."[14] Motivated tacticians are sexy, stable, and can be quick when you want them to be. He's someone who understands how to consciously control his cognitive unconscious, and he sees, most of the time, how and when he runs into attribution errors, cognitive biases, and shifty algorithms.

In short, you want to be like Max. (And it wouldn't hurt to marry a Max, either!)

TRUTH TAKEAWAY: In life, you want to be the person who finds the middle ground, learns how to leverage what works and what doesn't, and is curious enough to know you don't know everything.

Your cognitive unconscious is both really smart and really lazy. It's working a trillion operations at once (ones it's deeply memorized), and it would be cool with never learning how to work a new one again. This is where you come in.

Explore this list of biased ways your brain thinks about, perceives, judges, and interprets your world, your reality.

The Fundamental Attribution Error: Imagine you see a driver honking and upset in traffic. You might assume they're a jerk with road rage without considering that they might be rushing to the hospital to see their sick mother. This means you're relying on an internal attribution (personality trait) rather than an external attribution (the situation at hand). We tend to do this a lot: attributing the behavior of others to internal factors while underestimating the influence of external ones.

We judge other people in vacuums. But, as shown next, we treat ourselves as *only* products of our environment.

The Actor-Observer Bias: Suppose you forgot to do your chores at home one day; you'd likely attribute it to being too busy or distracted (an external attribution). But if your child forgets, you might call them "lazy" or "irresponsible" (internal attributions). We attribute our own behavior to external factors (like circumstances or pressure) while attributing others' behavior to internal factors instead.

We get the grace; they get the blame, and sometimes the screaming and the hitting. Not cool, parents (and also, abusive).

Why? Because your cognitive unconscious experiences what's called *perceptual salience.*[15] Perceptual salience occurs when you hold your consciousness flashlight in one spot of your warehouse or one spot of your external environment. What you focus on, what your attention is placed on, determines how you prioritize the variables you're working with.

When you're committing the fundamental attribution error while focusing on the behavior of someone else, *they* are where your flashlight is shining. So, *they* are the variable you attribute to the situation. It's their fault.

For the actor-observer bias, the flashlight is on the pile of your incomplete chores, an external situation. Therefore, your brain chooses a *situational* (external) variable as the cause instead of you. It's not your fault.

Some studies show, however, that when you initiate an experiment where you make people complete an activity similar to my Third-Person Mirror exercise from Chapter Three, the attribution of blame switches back to being internal, even if it's still about the external chore list.[16] When you see your own face, especially while doing something you're not happy or proud of, it makes you think about yourself and your situation differently—literally.

> **MAKE IT SIMPLE:** Your brain tends to find ways to blame others and release yourself from blame. It does this by quickly placing your attention on what it wants to blame. But, when you go face-to-face with yourself, you can grow in beneficial ways.

The Representativeness Heuristic: In addition to incorrect attributions, your brain also acts as an unconscious cognitive miser by using heuristics—mental shortcuts that take potentially complex judgments and problems and turn them into simple assumptions and solutions, even when they're not. Let's look at an example.

You just walked past a person who was wearing a tie, carrying a briefcase, and talking about stock market investments. It's easy to quickly assume he's a banker, right? This is an example of the representativeness heuristic at play. Your judgment is based on how closely he matches your mental stereotype of a banker rather than considering other possibilities, like him being a university professor who just lost all his money in crypto and is wishing he had stuck to a more traditional way of growing his money.

We tend to judge the likelihood of an event based on how similar it seems to a "standard" mental representation in our brains rather than considering other, more complex probabilities. We stereotype and categorize people, innately, whether we like it or not. And when we know better, when we admit more, we do better more often.

The Availability Heuristic: After seeing a news report about a shark attack, you might become overly concerned about shark encounters while swimming at the beach, even though the actual risk of a shark attack is very low compared to other dangers, like drowning or car accidents.

Another example: Consider a situation where you're planning a vacation. You recently watched a documentary about plane crashes and read a news article about a rare travel-related illness. Even though these events are statistically unlikely, the vividness of these recent and emotionally charged stories makes you feel that flying is a risky way to travel. As a result, you decide to take a long and exhausting road trip instead of a quick and safe flight.

Stop letting your cognitive unconscious mess with your vacations. Remember this heuristic. The easier you can recall or retrieve information from your memory, i.e., the more available it is, the more likely you will base your decisions on that information. You remember things more when they are emotional or recent.

The Anchor and Adjustment Heuristic: You're shopping for a new phone. The first phone you see costs $1,500 (how did we get here?!). This initial price is your "anchor." All the other phones, the ones for "just" $1,200 or $1,000, seem like better deals in comparison to the anchor, right? Yeah, if you're playing around with a budget like that to begin with, probably. Now, because of your anchor, you might be willing to spend more money than you originally intended because any adjustment of the price, lower than the anchor, appears to make the price more reasonable. (But I ask you again: Do you *really* need it?)

Label and learn your anchors—your initial value points (not just monetary values)—and make sure they're a reference point you want to be starting from. For example, do you consider someone a good friend just because they don't act like that horrible friend you had in high school or college? Or have you already restructured your idea of a friend over the years because that prior anchor wasn't an effective value point for you? (See how much work there is to be done?)

The game of "Fuck, Marry, Kill" might seem worlds apart from psychological social cognition theories, but in reality, they both involve making judgments and decisions.

Charlie, the cognitive miser; Nina, the naive scientist; and Max, the motivated tactician, each represent ways your brain can and does work at varying times. We can't simply "kill off" our cognitive unconscious (and its errors, biases, and heuristics) like we can Charlie, nor should we want to—they're vital for the game: the one in this book, and the one called life.

Rendezvousing with Nina every now and then—overanalyzing when, where, and how much you're making or potentially making unconscious cognitive decisions—isn't the worst idea. You may get more of your needs met. But, remember: Max, the motivated tactician, is and will always be the wisest decision.*

Your Brain Remembers More Than You Do

Your brain implements biases and heuristics (and even makes errors) by using past information and experiences when making its guesses. Therefore, it needs *memories*.

In your brain, you have the ability to form short-term and long-term memories. Short-term memory, often referred to as working memory, temporarily holds information relevant to your current ongoing tasks, like remembering a phone number while you find a pen to write it down. Short-term memory is exactly what it sounds like, memories held for a small burst of time so you can get something done.

On the other hand, long-term memory has a vast storage capacity (think of the warehouse again) and can retain information for extended periods, ranging from days to a lifetime. You have two types of long-term memory: explicit and implicit.

> **KNOW YOUR TERMS:** *Explicit* means active thought and awareness while *implicit* means unconscious or automatic information.

---

* Yes, my husband's name is Max. And yes, I'd say he is a motivated tactician . . . most of the time. He can also be a Charlie. I'm a mix of a Nina and a Charlie—and I pretend it makes me like Max. It kind of does.

Explicit memory involves facts, events, and knowledge that you can easily recall and articulate—things like numbers and facts, and personal experiences, such as your first day of school or a memorable vacation. It's easy for you to remember your explicit memories.

In contrast, *implicit* memory operates unconsciously. It includes things you don't have to think about to get done and things your brain automatically does for you, like your how-tos (driving a car, tying your shoes), priming (when you experience something and it affects subsequent thoughts or actions—like if I say "doctor," your brain might prefer the word "nurse" next instead of the word "table"), and classical conditioning, where your brain can learn to associate one thing with something else objectively unrelated—like not liking a song anymore because it was playing when you found out terrible news.

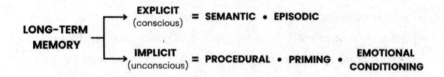

Implicit memories are a product of your cognitive unconscious. These memories form through repeated and/or emotionally important experiences and often guide your behavior without you realizing it. This can be a good thing or a not-so-good thing.

Sometimes, implicit memories can be helpful. For example, I once had a client who reconnected with her father for the first time in fifteen years. She had only known him up until she was eight years old, and many of those memories were suppressed or written over. Her brain didn't recognize him physically (for obvious reasons), but the moment he spoke, she broke down into tears and ran to hug him. Her somatic unconscious remembered the emotions her body felt around him—love, comfort, safety—and her cognitive unconscious stored that bodily feeling alongside the implicit memory of his voice. Her body stored the safety and her brain held her father's voice and that feeling of safety in the same place. *They* remembered him, even when *she* couldn't.

There's also a dark side to these hidden memories. Traumatic experiences can create memories that haunt us, leading to flashbacks, nightmares, and emotional pain. These memories can shape our views without us knowing it.

For instance, if we've had a negative experience with a certain group of people, our brains might make us feel uneasy around others who look like them, even if we don't want to feel that way. Your *unconscious* will decide how you're supposed to feel, think, and act around people instead of you consciously evaluating the situation and/or the individuals yourself.

These hidden memories can also push us to do things we might not want to do. If you have memories linked to addictive behaviors, like smoking or overeating, your brain might push you to do these things even when you're trying to quit.

Here's the big difference to remember: Explicit memory involves the *experience* of recall, when you're actively trying to think about things. Implicit memory is more like "remembering without remembering." It's sneaky, doesn't use words, and can be about how you act, feel, or sense things. For example, hopping on a bike and magically knowing how to ride it, that's your implicit memory in action—you don't have to think about it, you just start pedaling. Now, try to remember who first taught you how to ride a bike or drive a car or do any step-by-step task you've now memorized? That's explicit memory—when you *actively* remember something that happened.

Your earliest memories are going to be implicit because up until around the age of two or three, your brain was not developed enough to store explicit memory. Explicit memories require your brain to be more mature so it can store things better and use language to make things make more sense. We don't tend to learn to talk coherently until we're around three years old, which means our brain doesn't, either.

But it's not just infantile childhood memories that become the implicit memories our cognitive unconscious uses to direct our lives. I mean, we didn't learn how to drive a car or memorize the words to Vanessa Carlton's "A Thousand Miles" when we were one year old, but many of us somehow found the ability to do both simultaneously without really thinking about either one at least once in our lives.*

Implicit memory relies heavily on your unconscious—again, you "remember but don't remember." Since it's not something you use consciousness to tap into, you tend not to attach time to it, and it feels like it's happening right now, in the present. Why? Because time is a conscious construct. Implicit memories are the ones that feel like they're happening in real time when you think about them (for better or worse). When you jump on a bike and just start riding, it's like the bike was a trigger for that memory of riding a bike. It starts the same way as it did when you first mastered it.

And, when you get triggered by something that activates a traumatic implicit memory and behavior, it could turn into a complete and utter disaster, making your current moment in time feel like an upsetting time from the past where you need to defend and/or protect yourself.

Implicit memories can form through a variety of experiences and processes. Repetition is a key factor; when you repeatedly engage in an activity or experience something, your brain gradually forms implicit memories related to it.[17] For example, practicing the guitar daily can help your brain and body know exactly where you should put your fingers and the pick at the same time, eventually without thinking about it. This is how rock stars are made.

Strong emotions also contribute to implicit memory formation.[18] Traumatic events often create implicit memories that can trigger intense unconscious emotional responses. Conditioning, as seen in Pavlov's famous dog experiments,[19] is another path to implicit memory. Neutral stimuli become associated with involuntary responses, and over time, these associations become implicit. For instance, if someone you're interviewing for a job position is wearing the same cologne your ex wore, depending upon the outcome of your past relationship, you could be

---

* Can you hear the piano? You're welcome.

influenced to either like the candidate more or feel more inclined to reject them.

Sensory experiences, social learning, and cultural norms contribute to implicit memory as well—the unconscious memories in your brain are not just the traumatic ones. While they might stay hidden, implicit memories are always at work, silently guiding your actions, emotions, and perceptions throughout life. The strategy to bypass this would be to take time to reflect on your cognitive unconscious, see what may be coming up implicitly, and then redirect your decision to be based solely on the person's qualifications and the needs of the position.

We Are All Sheep

Let's look at three article titles:

1. "Democratic Voters Are Sheep."[20]
2. "The Sheer Hypocrisy of Republicans Referring to Democrats as Sheep."[21]
3. "Which Party, Democrat or Republican, Has the Most Sheep?"[22]

Let me answer number three: Neither party has more sheep. They're all sheep. We're all sheep.

Why are we talking about sheep—an animal known for following one another?

In late April 2017, Merriam-Webster added a new word to its dictionary: "sheeple" or "people who are easily influenced."[23] The example sentence they used was:[24] "Apple's debuted a battery case for the juice-sucking iPhone—an ungainly lumpy case the *sheeple* will happily shell out $99 for."[25] Urban Dictionary—an online dictionary for slang words—defines sheeple as "People unable to think for themselves" and "Those with no cognitive abilities of their own."

From the arenas of politics to technology to now the cognitive unconscious, people have been calling other people "sheep," or the combined "sheeple," for at least the last eighty-five years.[26] And we've done it so much it's now become a part of our permanent language.

What's most interesting is that this behavior of following, mimicking, and being influenced by others extends beyond our use of the term "sheeple." It's a fundamental aspect of human behavior and is deeply rooted in our cognitive unconscious. Obvious signs of this include observable behaviors like a baby smiling when a parent does (or vice versa) and people yawning when others yawn.

We often unconsciously mimic the actions, behaviors, and even emotions of those around us, experiencing what psychologists call emotional contagion and behavioral mimicry. We all blindly follow others—just like sheep.

Emotional contagion happens when emotions are transmitted from one person to another—unconsciously, and **behavioral mimicry** is the phenomenon where people often imitate or mimic the behaviors of others, also without conscious awareness.

Consider the power of social movements and protests. When a group of people gathers to advocate for a cause, their passion and determination can be contagious. Others who may have been indifferent or unaware of the issue can quickly become engaged and join the cause. However, these individuals usually don't choose to walk along the protest or scroll through people's social media content, saying, "I am going to go, and I'm going to look, and I am going to be persuaded!" (This is why advocates say even one voice matters, because that voice could be the one, perhaps the only one, that another person unconsciously latches on to.)

Ever watched a sitcom with a laugh track? These recorded audience reactions serve as cues for viewers at home to laugh along with the jokes. Even if you don't find a particular joke funny, the laughter of the audience can trigger genuine laughter from you.

Or what about stock market behavior? When panic sets in due to a sudden drop in stock prices, it often triggers a contagion of fear, prompting more investors to sell. Conversely, when the market is on an upswing, and people see others making profits, this can lead to a contagion of greed, driving more people to invest.

When you see people around you making decisions or feeling certain emotions—like deciding to drink alcohol or getting upset or angry—and you feel like you're stuck, wobbling back and forth between what to do, in these moments, you're actively battling between your unconscious and your consciousness. (Wild to think you've been in this battle your whole life and may not have known it, right?) Your brain is trying to make the decision for you, and you're trying not to let it.

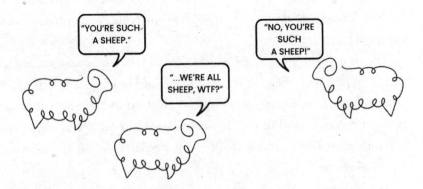

Understanding how your brain uses mimicry and contagion is crucial for your mental health because these processes can have both positive and negative impacts on your well-being. Emotional contagion can be a force for good when it comes to social support. When we witness others expressing empathy, kindness, or compassion, we're likely to mirror those emotions.

Unfortunately, contagion can also have dire consequences. In the context of mental health, individuals who are already experiencing emotional distress or mental health challenges may unconsciously "give" their emotional states to others, leading to the spread of negative emotions within social networks. Suicide contagion is a well-documented phenomenon where exposure to suicidal behaviors or suicides within a community can lead to an increase in suicidal thoughts and attempts among others.[27] However, and let me make this very clear, conversations about suicide with someone who is suicidal do *not* automatically increase the likelihood of them engaging in self-harm. Please continue to speak up and check in with those you love.

Similar to contagion, behavioral mimicry can lead to the adoption of helpful or unhelpful, adaptive or maladaptive habits. For example, if your friend starts going to the gym regularly, you might be inspired to do the same. Conversely, if someone in your social circle begins unhealthy habits like excessive drug use, you may follow suit.

You do what other people do. You are a "sheep" in some form or fashion when it comes to unconsciously following what other people are doing. Interestingly, these aren't the only times we humans engage in the act of blindly following. We also blindly follow what *our own brain* is already doing in two processes—priming, and situation and context.

Priming is the process by which exposure to one thing influences your response to another thing, without your knowing. The first experience plants a seed in your mind that grows into the next particular thought or behavior. Priming can take various forms, from visual cues to subtle suggestions, and it shapes your perceptions and actions more than you realize.

For instance, if you see images of elderly individuals, even briefly, you may unconsciously start walking more slowly, as your mind has been primed with the concept of "old age." Similarly, reading a news article about crime can prime you to be more cautious.

Understanding priming is crucial because it shows how your brain can be influenced by external stimuli, shaping your thoughts and behaviors without your explicit consent. Just as you often mimic and follow others unknowingly, priming shows how the world around you continuously shapes your unconscious responses.

And it's not just the real world that does this. It's also the world you imagine in your own mind. Studies have shown that just having an idea of something in your head, if it has enough commonly understood situational and contextual features, can affect you. The mere perception of a situation and its contexts in your brain can change how you act without your knowing it.[28] (And this isn't "manifesting"—that's a conscious action.)

In one study, researchers asked participants to deliver an envelope to one of a few various locations; when the location was a library—a place typically associated with quietness—without knowing it, the participants talked more quietly to one another while on their way than those with destinations other than a library.[29] In another study, participants were contacted via email over a weekend. Some were asked to describe their work office in a reply, some weren't. After the email portion, all participants were asked to complete a series of coin tosses and then report their "heads" score to the researchers—and they were playing for money. The more coin flips that landed on "heads," the more money they won.

The people who were asked about their work before the coin toss reported much higher "heads" tosses—way more than what would have happened by chance in comparison to the other group. Turns out, they worked at a bank. Thinking about their office—you know, the bank—unconsciously made them want to win more money, so they reported higher scores.

We may not like that we can be so easily and unconsciously influenced, but what studies have also shown is that we certainly *do* like it when others are seemingly influenced by us. In many cases, when people mimic *our* behaviors, we tend to not only tip them more,[30] but we'll also buy more shit from them and say we had a better time doing it.[31]

I'm Feeling Dirty, Give Him the Death Penalty

Imagine you've been offered two job opportunities.

One is a prestigious position with a renowned company, offering a high salary and a chance to attain prominent status in your field. The other job is less prestigious but brings home relatively the same amount of money and allows for a better work–life–family balance.

You initially decide to take the high-status job. Why? Because you're a human being, and you want to be successful in life. Success, to you, looks like career advancement and accolades (at least in this specific situation, it does).

However, after accepting, you find out that your partner has developed a mental condition that will benefit from having their family (you) more available rather than less.

It's safe to say that under these conditions, there would likely be some type of internal cognitive and possibly emotional battle.

Do you take the status-increasing position, convincing yourself that status leads to a better ability to care for your family? Or do you maneuver your way into thinking that it's best you take the more balanced job and ignore your desire for vocational recognition?

What do you do, what do you *want* to do, and why?

While there are many factors that will affect your decision-making, one major aspect of you as a human being that plays into every choice you make (this one included) is that within you, within all of us, are *fundamental human motives.*

Fundamental human motives[32] are deeply ingrained evolutionary drivers that influence your behavior. Whether you like it not, you're a human, and humans like safety, avoiding diseases, having alliances, gaining status, finding (and keeping) a mate, and taking care of one another. These are your human motives, and they control you both consciously and unconsciously.

When motives become active within you, certain parts of your body and brain—like your nervous system, your cognitive skills, and your language abilities—begin working together to meet the desired goal of the motive. These parts working together are called a "system." These motives, and their systems, have evolved over millennia to enhance the survival and reproductive abilities of us as a species.

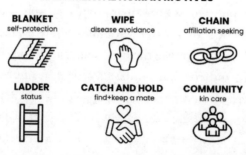

FUNDAMENTAL HUMAN MOTIVES

BLANKET
self-protection

WIPE
disease avoidance

CHAIN
affiliation seeking

LADDER
status

CATCH AND HOLD
find+keep a mate

COMMUNITY
kin care

Here are six fundamental human motives and examples of what may trigger them within you:

1. **The Blanket (*self-protection*):** The self-protection motive within you developed over time due to threats from fellow humans and other dangers. Its system and parts involve things like the fight-flight-freeze response, the ability to scan subtle and sudden movements, and the decision to make what seem to be safer choices. It's triggered by things like angry expressions, darkness, and scary situations. It acts like an internal security mechanism. When triggered, it heightens your awareness of potential threats and encourages, often without your awareness, cautious, risk-averse behavior or defensiveness and protection (in many varying forms).

2. **The Wipe (*disease avoidance*):** Disease avoidance evolved due to, as one would guess, the constant threat of infectious diseases. Think of this as your body's antivirus software. It detects cues related to diseases and prompts you to take actions to avoid contagion—such as initiating the emotion of disgust within you or making you consciously or unconsciously avoid unfamiliar or "dirty" environments, actions, or people, like when you move away from someone who smells *first*, and *then* have the thought, "Wow, that person smells" *second*. This usually happens so fast you don't realize the movement came before the conscious thought, but it did.

3. **The Chain (*affiliation seeking*):** The affiliation system traces its roots to your ancestors, for whom group living was essential for survival. It's your social network manager, one who uses parts of you—like the ability to read body language, social bonding hormones, and your ability to engage in cooperative-like actions—to influence your behaviors. It motivates you to seek connections with others and responds to triggers related to group dynamics, friends, and other connection-based markers.

   Now, your unconscious brain wants to keep you alive. So while you have an affiliation-seeking system inside you, your protection system will override this one if others have hurt you. The Blanket will keep you safe in isolation, and the Chain will make that safety feel deeply lonely.

4. **The Ladder (*status*):** Humans have a strong drive for status and a desire to gain respect and prestige in their social groups. When activated in you, the Ladder influences behaviors related to dominance, prestige, and competition by using your ability to perceive social hierarchies, feel envious or jealous, and your ability to buy status-symbolizing material items.

   This is a major system that becomes dominant in people with large egos (or small ones masked by defenses).

5. **The Catch and Hold (*find + keep a mate*):** Your mate acquisition system motivates you to seek romantic partners, is activated by cues of attractiveness, and encourages you to stand out. When you're seeking to "catch" a mate, this is the system that tells you you're attracted to someone and causes you to begin certain grooming or communication behaviors, to help you reach that goal—like moving your hair behind your ear or taking down your sunglasses to check the person out.

   This is your brain helping you connect more with the other person via sight and sound. There's no other reason for you to show your eyes or clear your ears. However, instead of seeing it as your unconscious showing, you just see it as "flirting." (This begs the statement: Just because you weren't "meaning to flirt" doesn't mean your brain wasn't trying to "catch" them.)*

   The Hold, the second half of this system, helps you maintain any existing romantic bonds you've already caught by guiding you toward things like being vigilant of others who may be interested in your partner, buying material items marketed toward relationship stabilization, and affectionate advances toward your significant other, e.g., getting jealous,

---

* If your partner is upset because you were "flirting" (and you actually weren't trying to), stop for a moment and talk about it. We're all human. Learn, and teach your brain. You don't need to separate because of it.

buying flowers or a watch, and giving hugs and kisses to your partner.

6. **The Community (*kin care*):** The kin care motive isn't responsible for making us have children (the Catch and Hold takes care of that by driving our desire to reproduce). Instead, kin care motivates us to ensure that those who need help get the care and attention they require—hence naming the motive the Community instead of something like the Children.

   This system encourages nurturing behaviors by releasing hormones, pushing you toward cooperative decision-making, and initiating nurturing behaviors. It's triggered by situations related to family, similarity, cohabitation, common goals, and even words like "brotherhood" or "sisterhood."*

So, basically, you, being a human, like being safe, disease-free, seen, respected, liked, and loved. And because you like these things, you make decisions that will lead to them. But that sounds too simple. Right? Yes, it does. Because it is.

> **TRUTH TAKEAWAY:** There is absolutely nothing wrong with wanting to feel safe, be secure, receive attention, gain respect, achieve success, and desire connection and love. It's human, and anyone who tells you otherwise is an asshole.

Fundamental motives aren't as direct and logical as they seem. It's not as straightforward as choosing a high-status job because you desire status or a family-oriented job because of family values. These motives can be, and very much are, unconscious and metaphorically utilized by your brain. For example, if you're a jury member discussing the punishment for someone who committed a crime and you're debating in a

---

* This is likely part of why that movie called *The Sisterhood of the Traveling Pants* was so popular. Traveling pants? No clue what that means. Sisterhood of them? Hmm, okay, tell me more.

dirty room, the mess might activate your Wipe system—unconsciously making you want to be clean and disease-free. This motive could cause you to suggest a stricter sentence for a crime—thinking of the crime or the individual as "dirty" themselves[33]—compared to a jury who deliberated in a clean room.[34]

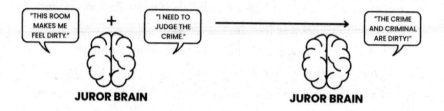

Your general disgust toward one thing (like dirt or foul odors) can become your embodied moral judgment toward something else—unconsciously. This is often why you see people who are racist or bigoted use the concepts of "dirty" people or "smelly" body parts to strengthen the negative perceptions of certain groups of people. (See, there's a reason I used the word "asshole" to make my last point.)

The example I gave in Chapter One about women who were looking at a dating site is equally disturbing. By activating their Catch and Hold system, the dating site changed their views on health behaviors like diet pills and tanning products from more negative and risky *before* viewing the site to more positive and less risky *after* viewing the site.[35] Our own personal values and beliefs can and do shift based on what's present (or recent) in our unconscious brain, like the last website we went to or the last influencer's profile we looked at.

The motives within you can be activated by external or internal cues. Using the Catch and Hold—the mating motive—as an example, an internal cue would be something like the ovulation phase of someone's cycle (which may prompt them to dress more "attractively" without knowing it), and an external cue would be something like seeing someone you find attractive and deciding to go up and talk to them. These examples may seem simple, and perhaps self-explanatory, but it gets more complex.

Once a motive has been activated, it changes what your preferences are and the choices you end up making at the end of every decision point in your life. And your motives can clash with one another, changing how you prefer to judge, perceive, and behave.

A need to protect yourself may lead you to conform to a group, but the desire for a mate may make you overcome your fears and stand out from the crowd—cue any episode of *The Bachelor* or *Bachelorette* ever. Combine (1) the framework around motives unconsciously influencing our decisions with (2) the fact that our brains are biased and lazy when it comes to assumptions, blame, and beliefs, and (3) mix in some alcohol, and those shows become a real-life depiction of the cognitive unconscious in human form.

Recognizing these motives will help you better comprehend your behaviors and motivations, offering insights into why you make certain choices, even when they seem counterproductive or irrational—like investing in a whole new wardrobe to impress that friend of a friend you were trying to get with but now they're with someone else, and you're out hundreds of dollars; or why you'd buy a bunch of organic household products after joining a workout club because that's what the "cool crew" is using to clean their house, even though you couldn't give less of a shit about "going green."*

Unacknowledged, unmet, and, most importantly, unconscious fundamental motives can lead to inner conflicts, stress, and emotional distress. By identifying and addressing these underlying drivers, you can achieve a better balance in your life, make healthier choices, and enhance your overall mental well-being.

Just as your memories can be implicit or explicit, so can your fundamental human motives, pushing and pulling you toward or away from certain thoughts, perceptions, judgments, decisions, and actions.[36]

---

* Hey, some people simply do not care about the planet. Don't shoot the messenger.

The Difference Between Emotions and Feelings

If you can't already tell, your unconscious is complex.

Everything about mental health and being human is *deeply* complex, which is why therapists are so misunderstood. Most people, even those with a positive outlook on the therapeutic process, think we do something as "simple" as "listen to people talk." Therapists are not passive listeners; we're interpreters of the unconscious messages you transmit as you talk, move, and share your understanding of life with us. Our task is to help you decipher as much of this hidden language as possible and then develop a plan with you on how to change it.

In the therapy room, one question echoes more than any other: "How does that make you feel?" This deceptively simple question can trigger a range of responses. Some individuals break down because, in this safe environment, they can finally articulate what's been deep within. For them, it's permission to release. Others, however, respond with a disconcerting "I don't know," often accompanied by avoidant eye contact or eye rolls.

For some, it goes even deeper, with responses like, "I don't even know what a feeling is."

If you've ever felt that way before—confused about what a feeling is, or even confused about what an emotion is, or maybe at this moment you're realizing you didn't even know there was a difference between feelings and emotions—let me unravel the framework for you.

Your emotions, at their core, can be defined as your body's sensations combined with your brain's interpretation of these sensations. Simply put:

Emotion = Body sensation + brain interpretation.

Emotions have a dual nature. They can exist in two states, as can almost everything else if you're catching on: conscious and unconscious.

Unconscious emotions operate separately from your consciousness, shaping your thoughts, behaviors, and motivations. They are potent drivers—influencing your decisions and reactions without you realizing it.

Unconscious Emotion = Body sensation + brain interpretation _out- side_ of your conscious awareness or control.

An example of an unconscious emotion would be how you react in a sudden moment of fear.[37] Your heart will race, your breathing will increase or hold, your muscles will contract, and you might stop being hungry.* This somatic reaction occurs unconsciously and automatically.

On the other hand, conscious emotions are those you're acutely aware of. They are the emotions you can see build up throughout a powerful song and the ones that have stories that color their experience— like describing happiness through the scenes of your wedding night. They manifest as what we commonly refer to as "feelings." Your feelings are the conscious experience of your emotional states.

Antonio, the USC neuroscientist, puts it beautifully when he says, "Feelings occur after we become _aware_ in our brain of such physical changes [like the ones mentioned above]; only then do we experience the _feeling_ of fear."[38]

> **MAKE IT SIMPLE:** Conscious emotions are "feelings" you're aware of and can identify, like happiness or anger. Unconscious emotions influence your thoughts and actions without you realizing it, such as an automatic fear response.

Conscious fear occurs when you knowingly feel afraid, like seeing a snake and recognizing your fear. Unconscious fear happens without your awareness, like feeling uneasy in a dark alley without knowing why, as your brain senses danger even if you haven't consciously identified a threat.

You're referring to _conscious_ emotions when you say you _feel_ happy, sad, angry, afraid, or anxious.

Conscious Emotion, aka "Feelings" = Body sensation + brain interpretation _within_ your conscious awareness or control.

---

* Your body knows it doesn't need to eat something if it's in a threatening situation. Who needs a sandwich when there's a lion attacking you?

UNCONSCIOUS = BODY SENSATION + BRAIN INTERPRETATION
EMOTION
outside your conscious awareness of control

CONSCIOUS = BODY SENSATION + BRAIN INTERPRETATION
EMOTION
(*feelings*)
within your conscious awareness of control

The most fascinating part of emotions is that they are deeply connected to your memories. In fact, many of your memories are snapshots of your past emotional states—capturing what your body and brain were undergoing during life experiences, both big and small. Meaning every emotion you've ever felt, with or without choice, has been stored within you as "important enough to remember."

What you experience in your body and brain becomes what you experience in your mind.

What you feel, and what you think, create the reality you live in—one where you either can (or can't) change and control your life.

CHAPTER 4 SUMMARY

- You don't see reality as it is; you build it from body signals, what's around you, and how you think about it.
- Your cognitive unconscious handles most of your thinking, from simple tasks to tough choices. It works well but can be lazy and easily tricked or biased.
- Your brain remembers much more than you do.
- It's completely natural to blindly copy what other people do.
- Just thinking about different situations can change how you act.
- Hidden motives drive your choices and actions, even those that don't seem to make sense.
- Memories and emotions are inextricably linked, whether you like it or not.
- Emotions and feelings are not the same thing.

5

Who You Are Is a Concept

The Psychoanalytic Unconscious

January 10, 2019, was supposed to be just another day—a breather, really.

Seven years into my BPD recovery, my husband, Max, and I were now the parents of a ten-week-old son—a baby we worked hard to conceive after months of in-vitro fertilization.[1] I was neck-deep in the completion of my clinical psychology doctorate, and together, we'd self-funded and launched a mental health treatment center.

Yet, under the veneer of long-term, sustained achievement (both personally and professionally), we were struggling emotionally. We were sleep-deprived, on edge (because caring for a newborn is stressful), and grappling with the echoes of a traumatic birth resulting in an emergency cesarean, multiple blood transfusions, and a painful recovery period. It had been a long two and a half months.

Exhausted and yearning for a semblance of normalcy, we elected for our very first "parents' night out." It seemed like a way to reconnect again, even if just for a few hours. We went out for dinner and stopped at a brewery, toasting the life we'd finally built together.

The night started off fine, filled with a sense of accomplishment and emotional relief. It was a brief hiatus from the never-ending cycle of sleep-less nights and diaper changes. But as night fell, our concept of "reality" started to unravel. An argument broke out between us, amplified by alcohol and our raw, precarious unconscious states—ones that resembled our old patterns.[2] As the night progressed, we drifted from "new parents" (in our conscious minds) to humans who had been together for thirteen years and had plenty to argue about (in our unconscious minds).

The evening unraveled rapidly; we needed to separate for a few hours. I left for a friend's house a few blocks from our apartment, and Max returned home shortly before the babysitter was set to leave, each of us surrendering to the unsteady forces within us.

Next came Max's troubling texts, touching on issues that had long been buried under years of my recovery (and the vortex of our new life's minute-by-minute demands). The state he was in—upset and intoxicated—was allowing his implicit memories, his unconscious, to take hold. He wasn't himself, and it was clear something deeper was going on—gnawing psychological unrest, one we'd later identify as masked and suppressed post-traumatic stress disorder (PTSD), resulting from our relationship's first six years.

I'll admit: For the first several years of our relationship, I was disloyal, dishonest, at times erratic and explosive, and contributed to many difficult nights that we both wish never occurred. Ones where I called the police on Max when he didn't deserve it and did nothing wrong.*

That night, after our argument and his return home, Max made the call—a 911 call he never intended to make. He texted to informed me that he had, in fact, accidentally called the police, didn't remember if he said anything, and then immediately hung up. Why did he call 911? We still don't know. Nothing was wrong.[3] At the time, regretfully, I didn't think much of it. I should have, for many reasons.

Within two minutes, police cars were speeding down the street, past the kitchen of the friend's house I was in, headed straight toward my home. Max texted me again, "The cops are here. Help, please." I had no anger, just a visceral worry, a sudden weight of regret. "What if I hadn't left him?" The raw urgency of the situation hit me like a freight train.

---

* This is one of the hardest things in my life to admit. Sometimes, you put people through terrible situations, more than once, and you live the rest of your life trying to make up for it.

I leaped down the stairs, into the middle of the street, and ran the four blocks as fast as I could. I think I might have also waved a car down and forced them to let me into the back seat to drive me two of the blocks. (It really was an intense situation.)

His seconds-long 911 hang-up call spiraled into a full-scale nightmare. The operator initiated a wellness check—as they should have with the lack of information they were provided, if any at all. Upon arrival, Max refused to let the police into our home—or let them confirm any level of safety within.

The result? An eruption of consequences: more police, SWAT, barricades, canines, crisis negotiators—the kind of response you'd expect for a dangerous criminal, not a family home in turmoil. Our street morphed into a surreal nightmare landscape, and our home—the place we created for our family to be safest—was under emotional, psychological, and now enforced siege. To see armed police officers with their guns pointed toward your home, your husband, and your baby is a special kind of terror.

Finally, after hours of heart-pounding fear and a series of anxious moments and desperate texts, Max came out of our home, disoriented, emotionally unwell, but physically unharmed. He was arrested, handcuffed, and led away. Although all but one charge would eventually be dropped (they tend to leave on charges related to the mishandling of police interactions), the aftershocks of that night's events would reverberate through our lives for a long time to come. It was a hellish revelation, exposing not just Max's unconscious psychological vulnerabilities but mine as well.

As I entered our home that night, with my newborn and without my husband, it was as though I was stepping into a different world, one I didn't recognize. My somatic and cognitive faculties were struggling to make sense of it all. The hallway looked alien, the air dense. I checked on our baby, his crib now standing as an eerie testament to the night's events.* I picked him up, held him close, as if to shield him

---

* Our son's crib was against the front window of our home, where all the guns were pointed.

from the invisible but palpable currents of tension that still hung in the air.

I walked around the apartment, every step feeling like a mile. This was our home, yet it wasn't. The newly formed concept of "home" we had created over the last few years had been transformed, if only for a night, into a theater of our vulnerabilities, our psychological fragilities laid bare for the entire city—and us—to see.

Our unconscious was showing and in a big fucking way.

Your body and brain act as a bridge between the experiences you have in life and your **"mind"**—the part of you containing your feelings, thoughts, and consciousness. When someone says a person is "out of their mind," it usually means they aren't acting consciously. Instead, their actions are fueled by their unconscious.

As your brain processes information about what's happening in the present moment, it creates **thoughts** (ideas, images, beliefs) and feelings. However, your thoughts and feelings aren't just affected by what you're experiencing at any given moment. As your thoughts develop, they are influenced by past emotions, thoughts, and memories you already possess.

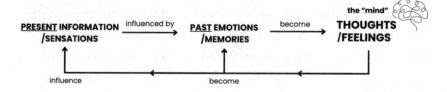

During Max's PTSD episode, his decision-making was mainly running on reflexes, and other unconscious past emotions and implicit memories. The recollections of Max's past became his present reality (this is what we clinicians call a flashback), and, in his mind, the past emotions and memories became so real his actions became delusional. But not the kind of delusional you're likely thinking about. You may be thinking about delusions as in wildly unrealistic beliefs, like someone who believes they are controlling the weather (which, as we can all agree, is factually impossible on a large enough scale for it to be recognized). A delusion is simply the belief in something that is not true. It doesn't have to be outlandish.[4]

> **KNOW YOUR TERMS:** Delusional: Believing in something false because of unconscious influences, even when you're faced with contrary facts.

Max wasn't "out of his mind," necessarily. He was instead "out of his *conscious* mind." As was I, completely missing the opportunity to be the supportive "wife" and "mother" I had worked so hard to become. In both circumstances, our unconscious was unknowingly making the choices we were *sure* "we" were making that night.

You may have noticed that I've placed several words in the introduction to this chapter and throughout this book in quotes, e.g., "reality," "bad," "home," "family," "mind," "wife," "mother," and there's good reason for it.

Eleven million bits of sensory information are sent every second from your body to your brain.[5] Eleven million! And your brain (well, the average human brain) can hold memory equivalent to 2.5 million gigabytes.[6] That's . . . a lot of input and a lot of storage.

Imagine all of this information—all these sensations, past emotions, memories, thoughts, and feelings—thrown into unorganized piles on shelves, all mixed together with no filing system or a way to easily sort through it, cluttered and lopsided all over your warehouse.

You pick up your flashlight to look around and feel massively overwhelmed. How are you, someone with extremely limited conscious ability (remember: your consciousness is weak, small, and time-restrained), supposed to try and make decisions—even unconscious ones—without sorting through all of this information? It would be an impossible task. (I get anxious even thinking about it.)

As you'd expect, your evolved human brain has solved this problem. As you experience life, your brain takes all the information you acquire and creates "*concepts.*"

Concepts are mental representations of your inner and outer world.

As a human, if you didn't hold concepts in your mind, you wouldn't have a clue what anyone was talking about. Nothing would be general. Everything would be specific. For instance, the simple word "hat" would not exist as a general term; instead, every hat in existence would require a unique identifier (like hat 1, hat 2, etc.). This lack of generalization would make everyday conversations near impossible, as you'd be forced to describe every detail of every object or idea you referenced.

It's super beneficial to have your brain unconsciously conceptualize things when it comes to things like fruits and cars and careers. It's not so helpful when it does it to people and behaviors—like conceptually placing a Black person into the category of "criminal" just because of the color of their skin, or assuming all people who use substances are "evil" because you smoked cannabis one time, thought you saw the devil, and couldn't handle it.*

> **MAKE IT SIMPLE:** Concepts streamline your thoughts and experiences by grouping objects, emotions, experiences (and, unfortunately, people) into broad categories. They're helpful at best, and limiting and harmful at worst.

Think of every concept in your mind as a specific area of your unconscious warehouse that you can explore, like wandering through the rooms of an IKEA. In each room, you find labels and tags placed throughout that uncover various elements linked to that concept— body sensations that you feel, memories that flash back, facts you know, perceptions you hold, and behaviors you exhibit, all tied to the concept you're contemplating.

It's like walking through the "living room" at an IKEA, feeling a soft couch, and seeing a TV, but, unfortunately for you, it's your concept of

---

* As a therapist, I can say, the human mind truly does conceptualize things in ways can be so incredibly damaging, to others and to ourselves, and for the wildest, illogical, righteous reasons.

"father" and you just feel fear and see those baseball cards he seemed to love more than you. *(Dark humor, apologies.)*

Another aspect to understand when it comes to concepts is that of **prototypes.** Prototypes are like the poster children of concepts. (Real quick: Remember when I started this book saying I was the poster child for what you'd consider being "out of control"? The only reason that made sense to you is because, in your brain, live your own personal concepts of "poster child" and "out of control." Your unconscious is always showing!)

Anyway, prototypes are the *best* examples of a concept—like when asked to think of a fruit, most people will think of an apple versus a pineapple, or when asked to imagine a pet, the most common image would be that of a dog or a cat instead of a kangaroo.

CONCEPT: fruit

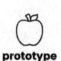

prototype   **prototype**

CONCEPTS

objects: fruit, ball
properties: red, small
abstractions: truth, love, hope
relationships: "worse than," "smarter"
intentions

Concepts and prototypes aren't just abstract ideas; they're an essential part of your daily life. You can find them everywhere, from the ideal "wife" or "boyfriend" to the idea of "mental health disorders" all the way down to the word "human," and which people are or are not afforded human rights. Concepts can be biased and fall into heuristics and errors (as you learned in the last chapter), or they can be nuanced, specific, and as accurate as desired or possible.

How *does* your brain decide what goes into these concepts and what doesn't?

Well, the answer is why this chapter exists: Your brain does its best, and often messes shit up. It does things you don't want it to do. It experiences your life and then decides that, against better judgment, it's going to conceptualize this new guy as your "ideal partner" because he acts like your ex but seems "nicer" (for now).

There's a reason why one of the oldest forms of psychotherapy is known as *psychoanalysis*. The word itself—psychoanalysis—can be broken down into two parts: "psycho" and "analysis." "Psycho" is derived from the Greek word "psyche," which refers to the mind. "Analysis" comes from the Greek word "analusis," which means to examine and analyze. When working with clients, the goal for psychoanalysts—clinicians who practice psychoanalytic psychotherapy—is an in-depth exploration of the concepts and processes within someone's mind—in their psychoanalytic unconscious.

The psychoanalytic unconscious is comprised of your mind's *experiential outcomes*—meaning the ways in which your life events have shaped you that you're not consciously aware or in control of. It's the best-known aspect of your unconscious and is called the "subconscious" by many. This part of your unconscious reacts to things like the pain–pleasure principle, counterfactuals (a fancy word for those "what-if" thoughts you always get), learned helplessness, and concepts like "bad vs. good," "pain vs. pleasure," "acceptance vs. non-acceptance," and "control vs. helplessness"—each of which we'll dive into in this chapter.

Your psychoanalytic unconscious is a dynamic part of you—where past and present intersect, shaping the narrative of your life and influencing your ability to feel in control, take the wheel, or remain a passenger. It's the part of me and Max's unconscious that almost fully took us over on January 10, 2019, when our family and the careers we had worked the past seven years for almost completely crumbled.

TRUTH TAKEAWAY: The hidden parts of your mind can shape how you act and react in life. Don't let predetermined concepts drive your decisions.

The Monsters in Your Mind

Think of the word "bad."

What is the first situation, object, or behavior that comes to mind? Based on what you've learned so far in this and previous chapters, ask yourself: *Why do I think this is "bad"?*

Is it because of personal experiences (like someone or something that hurt you in the past) or maybe it's because of societal and relational norms (where you've been told certain behaviors or objects imply certain intentions, morals, or values)? It's likely a combination of both.

Throughout human history, "bad" concepts like fear, shadows, the unknown, and darkness have consistently emerged. They represent not just our uncertainties but also the memories and thoughts we push away, both consciously and unconsciously. These "monsters" in our minds aren't just stories. They're deeply linked to your brain's structures, notably your **amygdala**—an almond-shaped cluster in your brain that unconsciously (and constantly) scans for threats.

Part of what challenges us as humans, aside from the difficult situations we often face without choice, is that our amygdala doesn't just affect our instant, natural fears. It also contributes to the development of learned fears or **fear conditioning**. Fear conditioning is a form of learning in which something neutral (like a blue square) is repeatedly paired with something hurtful (like a shock), until your body starts to act afraid of the neutral item or experience (where you are fearful of any blue square you see because your brain has linked it with the shock).[7]

Just like your emotions and your memories, your amygdala can also function consciously and unconsciously. Let me explain.

Your amygdala handles fear through two main routes: the cortical pathway, which taps into your brain's conscious, logical, thinking areas, and the subcortical pathway, which activates your unconscious, automatic responses.

> **KNOW YOUR TERMS:** Cortical: The outer layer of the brain, the cortex. Subcortical: Structures beneath the cortex.

When your amygdala takes the cortical route, it carefully analyzes situations to decide if there's really something to fear. When it doesn't, it reacts to your instincts, jumping to conclusions before waiting for a full analysis. Sometimes this is helpful, other times it's not.

When your conscious brain isn't fully engaged—maybe you're distracted, tired, or under the influence—your amygdala can misinterpret situations and trigger fear responses or defensive actions that are disproportionate or unnecessary, based on incorrect perceptions of danger. For example, seeing a mouse in a hallway may make you scream and jump as though it's a snake when you would have wanted nothing more than to be able to say, "No, that's just a mouse. Don't scream, you idiot, or you'll scare the caterer and they'll drop the cake!"

Your memories, particularly emotionally charged ones, are deeply influenced by your amygdala. When an event holds emotional weight—be it trauma, extreme joy, or anything in between—it's going to leave a more vivid imprint on your mind. Such events often reside at the forefront of your memory, easily accessible and regularly relived, whether you wish to relive them or not. Other emotional memories, our unconscious fragments and refuses to allow us to easily recall, if ever. These memories, your implicit memories, become the majority of your psychoanalytic unconscious.

And to top it all off, your amygdala doesn't only respond to threats it *actually* perceives; it's just as responsive to fears introduced via communication or instruction. A mere description of something scary, a cautionary tale, or even an overheard conversation can shape our fears. For example, a child might develop a phobia of bees, not due to a personal painful sting experience, but because someone graphically described the pain and aftermath of their allergic reaction. The concepts we come to fear in life—"monsters," "devils," "evils"—are profoundly influenced by our experiences and are controlled, in part, by the amygdala (a brain structure that seems to also, like many other things, have a mind of its own).

The concept of "bad"—those experiences, emotions, and parts of us that we hide away, perhaps even from ourselves—isn't new. But where does it come from, and how can understanding it help you?

We can't talk about the unconscious, fears, "bad things," and "monsters" without acknowledging the profound psychoanalytic insights of Freud[8] and Carl Jung—the Swiss psychiatrist and psychoanalyst who founded analytical psychology. Their theories provide a window into how we as human beings mentally process, conceptualize, contextualize, and sometimes suppress these conceptual fears.

We often hear terms like "burying our feelings" or "pushing down our emotions." Behind such phrases lies an old psychological observation that our minds, when confronted with distressing or undesirable thoughts, will actively push them into an obscure corner of our unconscious. Both Freud and Jung explored the territories of the mind beyond our conscious understanding, but their perspectives and conclusions varied.

Freud viewed the unconscious as a reservoir of memories, emotions, and desires, many of which he conceptualized as "unacceptable" or "unpleasant." He mapped out the human mind into three levels:

1. *Your Conscious Mind:* Your immediate awareness.
2. *Your Preconscious Mind:* Containing memories and thoughts which aren't immediately accessible but *can* be retrieved. (Think of it as a mental waiting room.)
3. *Your Unconscious Mind:* Houses memories and feelings that have been repressed due to being distressing or unacceptable.

Most people who use the word "subconscious" when referring to the part of their mind that influences their decision-making without their awareness are referring to the combination of Freud's preconscious and unconscious mind. However, Freud himself called these two aspects of the mind, when combined, the "non-conscious" mind.*

His second three-part theory was his model of personality. Freud's

---

* See . . . still not the subconscious. Why? Because, fundamentally, there is no part of your mind that is *sub*—or "below" another. Your whole brain and your whole mind are, in essence, always functioning at the same time. Sometimes you're conscious of it. Most of the time, you're not.

model of personality consists of the *id*, where your primitive desires reside (like your fundamental primary motives, except these aren't pathological or rooted just in sex or aggression as he believed), the *ego* (or your "conscious" self), and the *superego* (your internalized moral compass). Freud believed that a lot of your behaviors are just defense mechanisms, or strategies your mind uses to avoid confronting distressing thoughts or feelings—such as suppression (when you actively push down your fears) and repression (where your brain theoretically does it for you automatically).

Jung's take on the unconscious extended beyond the personal. He introduced the idea of the *collective unconscious,* a shared set of memories and ideas inherited from your ancestors. Central to this idea are **archetypes,** or universally recognized symbols, patterns, and concepts.

The four major Jungian archetypes are:

The Self: Which represents the unity of your conscious and unconscious parts.

Anima/Animus: Which holds the feminine side of men and the masculine side of women.*

Persona: The mask we wear in public—your persona will take on different forms based on your specific experiences, upbringing, culture, and general environment.

Shadow: This includes aspects of your personality you don't like, try to hide, or aren't even aware of; according to Jung, your biases and prejudices stem from here, and confronting and integrating your shadow is a crucial step in *individuation,* or the process of becoming the person you're inherently meant to be.

The monsters in your mind—your fears, suppressed traumas, and shadows—are a product of all parts of your unconscious working together. Your body senses, your brain responds, and your mind interprets, and they *all* remember. They *all* keep the score.

---

* Phew, lots of concepts in that line; society often forces us to suppress these opposing constructs within us.

Acknowledging your internal monsters (like the ones that emerged within Max and me the evening of January 10) is a necessary step toward consciously curating your unconscious. By understanding how your amygdala can unknowingly decide how you react to life (with or without actual fear) and combining that with the psychoanalytic insights of Freud and Jung—how we as humans tend to want to pretend bad things haven't happened to us and that we don't do or think anything that others wouldn't like—you can see and get to know your psychoanalytic unconscious.

In doing this, in seeing this part of your unconscious, lies the power to understand, confront, and eventually tame the conceptual "monsters" that reside within you. Are the "bad" things really there? Or does your amygdala just think they are? Are you really "bad," or is that conceptualization just based off someone else's life experiences that led them to tell you you're "bad" and you believed them?

Gremlin Playground

In 1996, the Sackler family, owners of Purdue Pharma, introduced OxyContin (a potent opioid pain killer), marking a turning point in the American opioid crisis. Their ambitious marketing strategies painted a picture of a life without pain, a promise that was irresistible to many, especially due to our human nature to seek relief from discomfort of almost any kind.

Unbeknownst to the masses, the Sacklers and Purdue were acutely aware of the unconscious and how it functions—in all three ways. They understood the intricate workings of the somatic unconscious and how the body doesn't like pain, the brain's unconscious cognitive mechanisms preferring quick and easy solutions, and, most importantly, the innate psychological human desire to imagine the rest of our lives going well, pain-free.

Central to the human experience are the pursuit of pleasure and the avoidance of pain, both physically and psychologically. This **pain–pleasure principle**, which operates unconsciously, is a driving force behind many of your actions and decisions. You, along with all people, naturally want to feel good and not bad. And the Sacklers used this instinct to promote OxyContin as the best new thing to hit the market when it came to "feeling better."

Their marketing campaigns were rampant and insistent. Physicians were wooed with lavish dinners (making their bodies feel good), conferences in exotic locations (giving them "good" memories linked with their brand), and monetary incentives (ensuring their brains thought of OxyContin before any other medication). The company sold the dream that OxyContin, with its timed-release formula, was a safer, less addictive alternative to other painkillers. However, and intentionally, they downplayed the risks.

The Sacklers capitalized on the fact that for humans, the allure of immediate relief, especially relief that promises newfound consistency and control, can be overwhelming. The unconscious desire to be free from pain, combined with a well-marketed solution that claimed "safety" was an irresistible combination for many. They exploited the human need for control over how we feel. Chronic pain can leave you feeling powerless. OxyContin's message was clear: You don't need to live in pain; you can take charge, and OxyContin will help you. This idea resonated deeply, especially within a culture that values autonomy and self-determination.

But as the years rolled on, the cracks began to show. Addiction rates skyrocketed, and communities across America were devastated by the opioid epidemic. Many users, initially prescribed OxyContin for legitimate pain concerns, found themselves dependent, and when prescriptions ran out, some turned to heroin and other illicit drugs.

In the end, it came out that Purdue Pharma had all the evidence suggesting the addictive nature of OxyContin but consciously chose to suppress it. The company knowingly played on the unconscious desire we have for relief and control, prioritizing profits over the well-being of patients.

I tell you the story of the Sackler family and their promotion of Oxy-Contin as a cautionary tale about how important it is for you to know how badly you unconsciously desire to seek pleasure and avoid pain. The Sacklers' control over this part of us as humans, combined with their disregard for the consequences, resulted in one of the most significant public health crises in American history, and you deserve to avoid the next one.

> **TRUTH TAKEAWAY:** Knowing how much your brain focuses on avoiding pain and seeking pleasure will help protect you from being manipulated by others.

Understanding how you function when it comes to pain and pleasure is a necessity for living as a human on this planet today. There is no escaping natural evolution, and you have evolved as an organism whose primary learning system for survival is, whether you like it or not, pain (and the avoidance of pain through fear).[9]

So you really get what I'm saying about the pain–pleasure principle, here's a helpful analogy created by Dr. Anna Lembke:[10]

GREMLIN PLAYGROUND

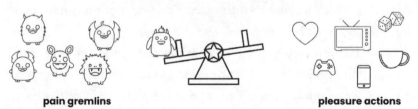

pain gremlins   pleasure actions

Picture a playground where you can see a group of children playing on a seesaw. When the children pile onto one side, that side goes down and the other side of the seesaw goes up, always in search of equilibrium. Similarly, your brain constantly seeks to find balance between pain and pleasure. When you experience a pleasure, it's like having all the children jump onto one side of the seesaw. Your brain tips to the side of pleasure, releasing dopamine (and other chemicals) to make you feel good. Dopamine is a neurotransmitter in your brain that plays key roles in pleasure, motivation, and reward. Chocolate, the laughter of a friend, a compliment, the touch of a loved one—these simple joys can cause your inner seesaw to tip toward pleasure. So can things like gambling, cheating, sex, drugs, and rock 'n' roll.

Here's where the analogy shows how messy this can be: Just as the seesaw strives for balance, so does your brain. After your pleasurable experience, your brain doesn't just return to its baseline. It now tips to the side of pain. When the children get off one side of the metaphorical seesaw in your brain, it immediately and at the same pace they exited shoots down the side of pain equal to the pleasure you just received. This pain might manifest as a craving for another piece of chocolate or a feeling of doubt when the compliments on your work stop coming in.

But what is it that forces the seesaw to rebalance itself? What unconsciously controls the pain–pleasure principle in your mind?

For the seesaw, it's physics. For your brain, as Lembke describes, these counterbalancing forces can be seen as "*neuroadaptation gremlins*" that hop on to allostatically (in response to your inner and outer environment) bring the balance back to your body, brain, and mind. The gremlins push the other side of the seesaw downward to "help" you.* **Neuroadaptation** occurs when your brain adjusts to the presence of something, often leading to tolerance or dependence on certain emotions, thoughts, or behaviors.[11]

So what if you keep feeding your brain pleasure over and over again? What if every time you felt a little down, you reached for another piece of chocolate or another dose of your preferred pleasure? Well, the gremlins will keep pushing down on the pain side, making it harder and harder for you to find balance, which will make you feel extremely out of control. (Which is a feeling you don't want and may label as "pain," which will in turn make you seek out more pleasure. See the problem?)

It's essential to recognize that not all pain is detrimental. Humans are hardwired to deal with pain; it's a tool for survival. Pain signals danger, teaching us to avoid it in the future. It's a learning tool, a guide, and a protector. However, in a society that markets endless solutions

---

* Even though that "help" can feel like the worst thing in the world, especially in circumstances of things like withdrawal from alcohol or grief when deep, deep love is lost.

for instant pleasure and relief from pain, we've begun to perceive any discomfort as unnecessary, as something to be immediately alleviated. We've lost the art of sitting with discomfort, of understanding it, and of using it as a tool for growth. Pain, in many ways, can be a teacher. If we allow ourselves to feel and process our pain, we can learn from it.

Now, this isn't to say you should seek out pain for its own sake, or that you need to experience certain types or levels of pain to learn lessons,* but rather that you should simply understand pain's role in your life, on a basic level. I want you to know that you register pain and pleasure as two ends of the same system. One does not exist without the other to you. And, therefore, you must be consciously aware of how your actions unconsciously influence the pattern of pain and pleasure seeking and avoidance in your life. (It's like I tell my clients engaging in harm reduction strategies: Use the drugs, don't let the drugs use you.)

> **MAKE IT SIMPLE:** Use pain and pleasure to your advantage. Don't let them take advantage of you.

When you exclusively chase pleasure, steering clear of any pain, you may unknowingly unbalance your mental seesaw. What starts as a benign craving for instant gratification can cascade into an insatiable need for more. Without equilibrium, the natural counteracting forces of your unconscious—the somatic, cognitive, and psychoanalytic—may plunge you into a cycle of compulsive behaviors and choices.

Your somatic unconscious, connected to your bodily sensations, will signal for more pleasure through physiological cravings. The cognitive unconscious, governing your automated thought processes, will justify these desires, telling you, "One more won't hurt," or "This is the easiest way to feel in control of my life." And the psychoanalytic unconscious, rooted in your deepest memories and experiences, might unearth past traumas and feelings to underscore the need for that hit of dopamine.

---

* Or whatever bullshit people say when you experience something traumatizing and they want you to "Find the reason behind it!"

True, the allure of a life devoid of pain is tantalizing. Yet, without challenges, how would we ever truly appreciate moments of joy, peace, and achievement? An uninterrupted life of pleasure becomes monotonous, lacking contrast and texture. I mean, think about it. Sure, monks seem content, but I've always thought their lives seemed a bit boring (no offense).

"What If" Things Were Different?

"What if I acted differently?"
  "What if I let them borrow my car?"
  "If only I said what I really wanted to say."
  "If things were different, they would not have lost their jobs."

Have you ever found yourself lost in thought, wondering how different choices in your past might have shaped your life today? What if you had made alternative decisions or had taken divergent paths? Maybe with a little more effort, you could have finished that degree or booked a date with that employee from your local store. Perhaps if you hadn't run through that yellow light, you could have missed the accident.

Thinking about what might have been, alternatives to our own past, is central to human thinking and emotion. These thoughts are deeply ingrained in our nature. If we could *only* accept our life experiences *as they happen*, with no capacity to wonder how they might have happened differently, we'd be permanently trapped in the present, unable to learn from our past or plan for our future. And our brains . . . would hate this.

As much as we're told to "be in the present," we also need to have, and are innately wired with, the ability to explore the what-ifs that linger in our minds—it's how we make sense of our experiences, learn from our mistakes, and prepare for uncertainty.

In the clinical and research world, we call these thoughts *counterfactuals*. **Counterfactuals** are thoughts that involve imagining alternative scenarios to past events or actions, exploring how things might have unfolded differently.

They happen in your mind in three steps.[12]

Step 1—Activation: You experience something—like not getting a job you applied for. This experience leads to the activation of a cascade of related and relatively important sensations and memories stored in your body and brain, like remembering how you confidently applied for this one, how you felt nervous in the interview, and all of the reverberating anxiety that's been living within you as days passed and you waited for a return call.

Step 2—Inference: Now, like a movie in your mind, you're playing scenes of how it could have turned out differently. You start exploring the what-ifs—what if you answered that question differently than you did? What if you were the first interviewee instead of the last? You're mentally changing how you see the actual experience, and this influences your emotional response to it. At the end of the inference, you ultimately decide that the reason you didn't get the job was because "*You* did *something* wrong."

Step 3—Adaptation: Once you've engaged in counterfactual thinking, depending on your locus of control (whether or not you believe your actions influence your outcomes), you'll use the insights you've gained to guide your future decision-making—maybe next time, you'll pick a different interview time slot, prep more by learning about the company, or memorize your answers less so you seem more relaxed. If thinking you did something wrong upsets your brain too much, it will find a way to push the blame off onto someone or something else.

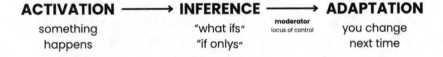

ACTIVATION ⟶ INFERENCE ⟶ ADAPTATION
something   "what ifs"   moderator   you change
happens   "if onlys"   locus of control next time

Understanding how counterfactuals can impact your life is important. You can, and likely do, use them to analyze, plan, and predict your past, present, and future, engage in creativity, and find meaning in setbacks.[13] And, like *everything else* you've learned in Part I, counterfactuals can be unconscious and automatic and can significantly affect and be affected by your life experiences—good and bad.

There are two different kinds of counterfactuals, and your brain will often automatically create specific counterfactuals under certain conditions.

The first is **upward counterfactuals.** These are the ones where you imagine how a situation could have been *better*—"If I received the alarming note sooner than I did, I could have saved them." They make us want to *be* better.

The second is **downward counterfactuals.** Now, these are the mood-boosters. They make us think about how a situation could have been *worse*—"I didn't even want a nighttime job; if I did get this one, I wouldn't have been happy." They're alternative realities to make you *feel* better.

When you experience a positive event, your brain automatically makes downward counterfactuals. In other words, when you're happy, your brain will automatically say: "It could have been worse." *Your brain wants you to stay happy.*

However, what your brain won't automatically do when you experience a positive event is help you get to an even more positive outcome. You have to *consciously* control your thoughts and say something like "Still, it could have been better." Meaning if you want to be motivated after success, you have to work hard at it. Your brain, already feeling positive about itself, doesn't care to put in any more work.*

When things are going well, it's a lot easier to keep yourself elevated and think about how bad shit *isn't* happening than to think about future good shit you *could* get if you were even better next time.

Conversely, when you experience a negative event, your brain automatically makes upward counterfactuals. Meaning, when you're upset, your brain will automatically say: "It could have been better." *Your brain wants you to learn from your mistakes.*

If you want to be positive after something negative happens, you have to consciously tell yourself things such as "It could have been worse."

---

* This is different than people who are never satisfied. Those types of individuals tend to not feel the initial happiness that comes along with this phenomenon.

When shit happens, it's a lot easier to be hard on yourself and think about what you don't have than to experience gratitude for what you do.

When it comes to the unconscious, motivation is harder than complacency, and regret is easier than acceptance; unless the goal is motivation rooted in regret or acceptance for the sake of complacency.[14]

For example, Olympic bronze medalists often feel more satisfied than silver medalists because of counterfactual thinking. While silver medalists think about how close they were to gold (upward thinking), bronze medalists are relieved they got a medal at all, rather than missing out (downward thinking).[15]

However, if you feel in control,[16] and if you have a good level of self-esteem,[17] you can turn things around. "It could have been worse" can start to become your unconscious response to negative events, and "It could be better" could become more automatic when things are already going well. The 12 Steps of Consciousness you're soon to embark on will help you feel more in control, and should boost your self-esteem, which means you'll also be reprogramming your mind's counterfactuals!

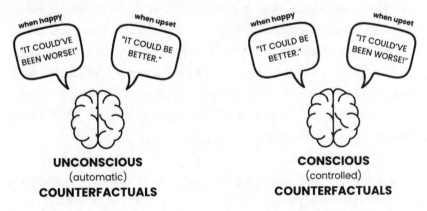

But wait, if your automatic counterfactuals can improve when you're feeling in control and good about yourself, then what can happen if you feel out of control and bad about yourself? And how does the fact that your brain continuously and automatically tells yourself that you should be complacent and regretful in life impact you?

While counterfactual thinking can be a powerful tool, it's also a double-edged sword. Comparing reality to what might have been can trigger a roller coaster of amplified feelings, from relief and satisfaction to anxiety and guilt.[18] It's not all sunshine and rainbows like your unconscious wants it to be.

When left unchecked, it can take a dark turn. Regret (something your unconscious is particularly good at) has strong links to depression and anxiety. Severely depressed individuals sometimes entertain counterfactual alternatives that appear unreasonable to others, intensifying their emotional struggles.

Traumatic life events can often trigger counterfactual thoughts as well, significantly impacting well-being. For example, those who lose loved ones in accidents and continue to dwell on what might have been experience greater overall distress. And the frequency of these types of counterfactual thoughts is linked with increased symptoms of PTSD.

Accepting life and saying statements like "Everything happens for a reason" or "It is what it is" is often seen as a noble pursuit, aiming to bring serenity in the face of life's challenges. But the reality is, our brains are not hardwired to simply accept everything. If we did, we'd gladly accept death; instead, your unconscious (the thing that makes up 95 percent of you) fights to use any ounce of control it can perceive to keep you alive.

Biologically, you're designed to be a problem solver, to evaluate situations, and to act in your best interest. While the concept of "acceptance" can offer comfort and a sense of peace, your natural instincts will most often push you toward action, reflection, or even resistance. Don't judge yourself for this. It's human.

> **MAKE IT SIMPLE:** Even though accepting things is important, we're naturally made to question and sometimes resist our situations. Refusing to accept something that is unacceptable is completely okay.

In practical terms, there are situations where passive acceptance isn't even beneficial or safe. For instance, accepting injustice without pushing for change can just perpetuate continued harm. Furthermore, just because we know it's often healthier to accept things we cannot change doesn't make the process automatic or easy. Our brains will always weigh, analyze, and sometimes challenge the reality before us, again, whether we like it or not. It's not a flaw; it's just how you're built. There are ways to make it easier. Part II will help, a lot.

You Don't Learn Helplessness, You Detect Control

In 1967, Steven Maier and Martin Seligman, two American psychologists, discovered a phenomenon they named "learned helplessness"— where, in certain situations, we learn that no matter what we do, it doesn't matter, and so we give up. Their theory was that, in essence, we "learn" we're helpless. Turns out . . . they were partially wrong; they admit it, and you need to read about it.

The following is essentially a summary of their "whoopsie-daisy" article that came out in 2016.[19]

In the early 1960s—a time when psychology research was shifting from behaviorism (the study of learning and modifying observable behavior) to studying more cognitive-type perspectives on how and why we function (i.e., what's going on in the brain that we can't directly observe)—researchers wanted to understand how *fear* could affect learning.

So Martin and Steven divided dogs into three groups. The dogs in Group 1 were simply harnessed and released after a period of time. The dogs in Group 2 received electric shocks but could escape them by pressing a panel. And the dogs in Group 3, well, they received the same shocks as Group 2, but had no way to stop them.*

The next day, they placed all the dogs in a shuttle box—a rectangular chamber divided into two compartments by a low barrier. When a tone was played, an electric shock followed, and the dogs could escape by jumping over the barrier to the other side. Dogs from Groups 1 and 2 quickly learned to escape the shocks by jumping over the barrier. However, most dogs from Group 3 did not attempt to escape. They just stayed there, passively waiting to get shocked.

Steven and Martin were confused: Why did these dogs not try to

---

* Sorry for the mental images or physical sensations that may come into your consciousness here.

help themselves? What happened next was a deep investigation into this phenomenon, a phenomenon similar to what we humans conceptualize as *helplessness*.

In their analysis, they considered two forms of helplessness: objective and subjective.

Objective helplessness happens when your actions simply don't change the outcome, like no matter how much you move, you aren't going to stop the shocks. Your actions don't matter, behaviorally and probabilistically. In the first part of the study, the dogs in Group 3 were objectively helpless. They could not physically escape the shocks.

On the other hand, **subjective helplessness** is about cognitively recognizing that your actions can't stop bad things. It's learning, *consciously*, the idea of and *knowing* that you are, in fact, helpless. In the second half, when the Group 3 dogs could escape but didn't, they were subjectively helpless.

The study seemed to show that the dogs who were objectively helpless also subjectively learned they had no control over their situation. They expected, after being out of control for as much and as long as they were, that they'd still be out of control and shouldn't try to do anything about it. It led them to the conclusion that the dogs in Group 3 "learned helplessness." It was the best explanation they could come up with at the time, considering the research tools they had access to.

Initial assumption: Uncontrollability (leads to) ➡ increased helplessness

After the dog experiments, Steven and Martin went their separate ways. Martin went on to study helplessness in human settings, found that how people *explained* and *described* their helplessness affected how long it lasted (remember this for Part II), and considered what the helplessness phenomenon could teach us about depression.

Steven moved into neuroscience and found through evidence in the brain that (1) being adversely shocked causes passivity and anxiety (not a shocking revelation), (2) detecting the ability "to control" prevents passivity and anxiety, and (3) "expecting control" leads to changes in the brain promoting action to avoid being hurt. In case that was confusing, Steven basically found out that getting hurt makes you freeze and get worried, when you think you can stop yourself from getting hurt it makes you freeze and worry less, and that expecting you can be in control makes your brain want to do something to avoid getting hurt.

By the 1990s, researchers had learned a ton of new information about how the brain responds to painful things—like shocks. They found specific parts of the brain that play a big role in how we react to stress and other feelings and sensations we can't control.*

Here's where they realized they needed to update their original idea: Later studies using advanced brain imaging techniques showed that both controllable and uncontrollable stressors activated certain parts of the brain. But there was a key difference in how long this activity lasted and which other brain areas got involved.

After shocks that couldn't be avoided, these brain parts remained active for an extended time, keeping anxiety and feelings of helplessness higher for longer. In contrast, when shocks could be escaped, and they *learned* they had control over the situation, the brain's anxious and passive responses decreased over time.

To make it simple:

It's not that lack of control leads to *learning helplessness.*

It's that *detecting control* leads to you calming down and trying to help yourself.

Secondary assumption: Perceived controllability ➡ decreased helplessness

So, now they had to learn about control (like what you're doing in this book) because *detecting control* seemed to be what *alleviated helplessness.*

Often, it's not helplessness that's learned, it's control.

By conducting more studies, they came to realize that if you exposed someone to escapable shock (a controllable situation) before exposing

---

* You don't need to know details on these brain parts, so don't worry; or, I should say, try not to.

them to inescapable shock (an uncontrollable situation), anxiety, passivity, and fear would be initially prevented or reduced during the second, uncontrollable situation. Experiencing controllable stress could actually protect against the effects of later uncontrollable stress—like giving your brain a workout in dealing with stress.*

But it's not just about controlling things in the moment; it's also about how we expect things to happen. When we experience control, our brains rewire themselves, expecting that we can handle future stressful situations. This can explain why sometimes we feel more in control and less stressed, even when things get tough—because we know, unconsciously, that we can handle it.

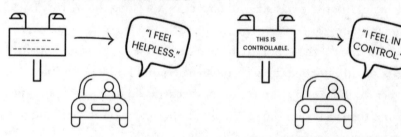

I want to stress the importance of how the basic detection of control can reduce your anxiety and alleviate helplessness. Not even the action of *being* in control, just knowing *you can be.*

In one experiment, people were asked to perform various mental tasks while a distracting noise played in the background.[20] Some of them had access to a switch that could turn the noise off. They barely used it, and they performed better than people who didn't have a switch. Just being consciously aware of *the ability* to control your life can sometimes be enough to reduce the impact of something getting in the way of your goals.

The human journey toward healing is profoundly entwined with our conceptualizations of "controllability" and "helplessness." We naturally yearn for a grip on our surroundings, our experiences, and, most criti-

---

* Remember this. The 12 Steps of Consciousness are stressful. But it's controllable stress. You'll see soon.

cally, our emotions. But this grip, this sense of control, isn't just about managing external factors. It's intrinsically tied to our self-perception and the narratives we've been fed throughout our lives.

Unfortunately, societal discourse often misattributes a person's feelings of helplessness to personal inadequacies, further cementing negative self-concepts. When society tells someone, "It's your fault you feel this way" (without giving them any way to do something about it), it's not just an external condemnation but it can become an internalized narrative of self-blame. The belief that "things will never get better" intensifies when one perceives a situation as completely and entirely outside of their control. This perception is not just cognitive—it's deeply emotional, and it taps into the primal regions of our brain responsible for survival.

Hear me when I say: You CAN consciously control and change your life. **You can.**

Even if you can't be in control of the one thing causing you the most pain in your life at this moment, there are things you *can* be in control of. Even if you want things to change that can't change, there *are* aspects of your life that are changeable, and **you can change them.**

Part I of this book taught you about your somatic, cognitive, and psychoanalytic unconscious. You participated in both thought- and experience-based exercises that showed you the conscious control you can have over your unconscious—like moving your attention onto the temperature of the air going in and out of your nose, watching how your mind quickly gets things wrong, and asking yourself why the first thing that pops up in your head when I say, "Think of something 'bad'" is actually bad. You now know subtle and general ways that your unconscious is showing. But the subtleties in life never really got anyone anywhere, at least not anyplace worth taking someone else to. Thus, it is now time for Part II.

In Part II, you will learn how to consciously control and change your life, using everything you learned in the first half of this book and by diligently completing the 12 Steps of Consciousness. The 12 Steps of Consciousness are a structured set of guidelines designed to help you achieve a higher level of self-awareness and therefore more control. They are designed to help you become a more conscious human being in the unconscious world you live in. Because, yes, it, too, is unconscious as fuck. Probably 95 percent unconscious, just like you are.

As I mentioned in the beginning of this book, we treat ourselves and one another terribly because we don't understand ourselves. So, each of the twelve steps builds on the previous one to not only deepen your understanding of yourself and your three-part unconscious, but to also grow your conscious connection to the world and the people around you.

We're going to hack what's hidden, reprogram what's automatic, and shine a light on and rearrange your warehouse.

Are you ready for it?*

CHAPTER 5 SUMMARY

- Your psychoanalytic unconscious holds past experiences and storylines that run your entire life.
- Concepts simplify life, but make you lose out on nuance and complexity.
- The monsters in your mind are made up and are very important.
- If you don't control pain and pleasure, they will control you.
- Accepting things is cool, but it's not what you're programmed to do.
- Often, it's not that you "learn helplessness," but that you detect control.

---

* Yes, I did mean that as a Taylor Swift reference.

PART II
THE 12 STEPS OF CONSCIOUSNESS

The 12 Steps of Consciousness

Step 1
Admit it: Your unconscious is showing and it's controlling your life.

Step 2
Believe there's a better, more conscious version of "you."

Step 3
Intentionally commit to consciousness as your tool for change.

Step 4
Look at the unconscious mess you've been avoiding.

Step 5
Get honest: Share your unconscious patterns with another human being.

Step 6
Prep yourself: Create a list of ways you want to curate your unconscious.

Step 7
Do the work: Consciously curate your unconscious.

Step 8
Take accountability: List the people your unconscious behaviors have harmed.

Step 9
Actively amend your unconscious interpersonal harms.

Step 10
Enlighten yourself regularly; unconscious patterns are powerful.

Step 11
Continuously expand and adjust your understanding of consciousness.

Step 12
Grown consciously? Good. Now, help someone else do the same.

6

Be a Human First

"Our unconscious is not more animal than our conscious, it is often even more human."

—Edward Bond, *The War Plays*

Let me set the scene:

It's nine months past the January 2019 incident. Max and I are getting lunch at The Big Yellow House Restaurant in Summerland, California—an unmissable restaurant with bright yellow paint peeling off its large exterior, directly off the 101 freeway. It's a place with screen doors, creaky steps, and an appropriate level of flies given the temperature and the overall vibe of the place. At one of the tables sit two quickly condensating plastic water cups, a basket of fries, and Max and I, holding hands across the table, looking into each other's eyes.

It's September 5, our anniversary—fourteen years to the day since the start of our high school sweetheart relationship, and the date of our wedding. I have two cards laid out on the table: one to share my overall thoughts on our journey out of the unconscious hellhole we accidentally opened earlier in the year and another to showcase my commitment to consciously loving the man who put so much effort into loving me, even through all my early years of primarily unconscious behavior.

Max opens and reads each card.

Card #1:

September 5, 2019

Dear Maxwell,

Since our last anniversary, we became parents. You've remained my husband, and I your wife.

I'm growing. You're growing. This is life. This life is important to me, as are you, and our son.

Thank you for who you are. Thank you for being someone with whom we can talk about the darkest things we've done, seen, and said in our lives, and we can hold them up into the light without a flinch.

I'm not afraid of our love, or life with our love in it. We're meant for each other.

I have no doubt that my soul knew you were the one from the moment we locked eyes.

I'm so proud of us.

Love, Your forever wife

Card #2:

This year, my gift to you is: MY SOBRIETY.

I've done a lot of thinking recently and I'd like to grow with you in ways impossible without full clarity. It is my decision to be 100% clear in this life with you for the next year.

I can't wait to grow with you and grow our family.

Thank you for your patience.

Two sentences stand out from the cards I handed Max that day, and they're particularly important for your upcoming journey through the 12 Steps of Consciousness:

1. "We can talk about the darkest things we've done, seen, and said in our lives, and we can hold them up into the light without a flinch."

This is vital for conscious growth. If you can't look at the monsters, the shadows, the concepts, biases, and patterns in your unconscious, they'll never leave. They'll never change. They'll always have the potential to control you, without you knowing it.

This sentence written to Max in Card #1 was *my* commitment to my own 12 Steps of Consciousness journey—the same one you'll embark on shortly.

2. "I'd like to grow with you in ways impossible without full clarity."

You do not have to be sober to engage in the 12 Steps of Consciousness. While they were adapted referencing the 12 Steps of various addiction groups like Alcoholics Anonymous, they do not address the need for and do not require sobriety. Remember, this is not about recovering from using substances, it's about recovering from *being human*—one with an unconscious yet to be thoroughly explored.

For me, dissociating from my physical body has always been a go-to coping skill.* And the quickest and most efficient way I know how to personally dissociate from my physical body is by engaging in substance use. For this reason, when I am actively and consciously working on myself, I abstain from using. However, I am not a fully abstinent human being and do not hold a standard that everyone healing and growing consciously needs to be.

For you, allowing yourself to grow with *full clarity* through this 12 Step journey might look different. Instead of abstaining from substances, perhaps you'd refrain from hanging out with a certain friend group, going to certain events or locations, or not engage in conversations with specific family members that just seem to upset you and make you feel like you're taking steps backward instead of forward.

When it comes to clearing out your body, brain, mind, and life to prepare for the steps required to grow consciously, you know what's best. You know what works and what doesn't work. *You just need to listen to yourself, your whole self, all your parts.* What do you need to

---

* Yes, I know, not the best one most of the time—I learned it very young, and for good reason.

remove, add, or change so that you feel more clear, capable, and willing to stay the course and not get thrown off? Take some time to think about this. As you've learned, your environment, both internal and external, conscious and unconscious, plays a major role in how you think, feel, act, and perceive.

I've spoken a lot in this book about how in order to grow and control your life you have to shine your conscious flashlight into your unconscious warehouse, look around, learn and unlearn some shit, and then do something about what isn't working. During the nine months between the big incident and our anniversary this day in Summerland, however, I had failed to take several of the steps you'll soon learn about.

Waking up on the morning of January 11, 2019, post Max's arrest, there were news cameras outside my front door, and Max's mug shot was plastered all over the local news channels (all cities need something interesting to talk about, and the police needed to explain the late-night commotion). I was hiding. Seven years of healing work and, to me, in those moments, all there was to show for it was me hiding myself and my newborn behind closed curtains while I cried—worrying when my partner would be able to come home. Traumatized. Scared. Alone. This was the life I tried so hard to avoid, worked so hard to not experience. This was the story of my mother raising me, a childhood for my child I wanted so desperately to avoid. I was not okay.

Instead of growing consciously, I fell . . . deep into my dark, unconscious warehouse. Picture Alice drowning in the sea of Wonderland. When my feet hit the ground, it was as if I started tossing all the storage file cabinets up in the air, pushing all the conceptual and perceptual aspects of my life off balance, essentially trashing the place. Convincing myself that this (this being: forever consequences of my past unconscious actions) is all there would ever be, and saying things to myself that I'd once heard said to me by others in my past: *"This is just the way things are, and how they always will be."*

In order to cope (inappropriately and maladaptively) I escaped to Vegas without notice, stayed out late with random town locals, numbed my body, brain, and mind, and allowed the negative stories about myself, my past, and my life to become my present. This is how I acted for the majority of my life before I started on my initial healing journey—the one prompted by Max's ultimatum. How did I end up here *again*? I needed to know why, and I needed to make sure it never happened again—I had a child's life in my hands now, and I know what it feels like to be a child struggling due to circumstances you have no fault in.

So, beginning this day, September 5, 2019, I decided to tell more of *the truth* to myself and others than I had ever been able to before. I had to. I needed to consciously curate my unconscious, especially if it was going to always be there. There was no way around it if I wanted to be sure I was in control of my own life.

I had to accept that while I had touched several parts of my unconscious on my healing journey already, I hadn't touched them all. Just like the blind men and the elephant, I needed to broaden my understanding of what I couldn't see in order to truly grasp all of my parts—conscious and unconscious.

I submitted to two big, hard truths that year (and began sharing them on my newly developed social media account, @the.truth.doctor, on my son's first birthday in late October):

1. My unconscious was showing (and it always would be); and
2. I am a human first (no matter what, even when it hurts—*especially* when it hurts).

Here's the interesting thing about these two truths: They're paradoxical in nature.

The more you admit your unconscious exists and controls you, the less power it has to ultimately control your existence. And the more you accept you're a fucking human being—one that struggles, is primarily unconscious, and isn't perfect—the less painful and shameful it is to be human. Put simply:

THE UNCONSCIOUS PARADOX

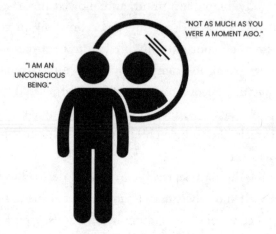

The more you accept your unconscious, the less unconscious you become.

And, the more you admit being a human is hard, the easier it becomes to be one.

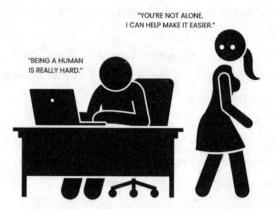

THE HUMAN PARADOX

Your unconscious is showing. It's showing in all human beings. There is no way around it, and it is all around us. When we forget this, we fall into the depths of uncontrollability, lack of self-esteem, the perception of lack of control, shame, blame, and many other ways we tend to curse our own existence.

As you walk the 12 Steps of Consciousness beginning in the next chapter, there are three things I want you to remember:

1. *You choose* what your journey is going to look like. You're done using a predetermined, unconscious blueprint designed for you by a world that existed before you did. You decide how radical or spiritual, major or subtle you want this to be. **You're in control.**
2. It's likely not your fault you are where you are, but *it is your responsibility* to move forward. Again, **you're in control.**
3. *You deserve to be self-conscious*, but not in the negative way you're thinking of in this moment.

What often prevents people from beginning their healing journey, kicks them off the positive path they're already on, or makes them decide they no longer want to heal and would rather self-destruct (like the decision I made in January), is feeling like they're doing something wrong, that they are completely out of control, and/or that everything is against them. But here's the problem: Almost everyone I know, my clients and myself included, who ends up finding themselves in this position (where healing "isn't possible" or we're regressing) is making this decision based off of blaming themselves for being *human*—for doing and experiencing completely normal human behaviors and typical, evolutionarily expected experiences.

We tend to judge people by the labels found within the mental health field. Something is "typical" and "normal" if it doesn't land on a symptom list of a mental disorder or condition. And if you *do* have a condition or a disorder, then it's as though you aren't allowed to have a normal human experience because *all* your experiences have become pathologized.

Let me explain using what I like to call my Salad Analogy.

Think about a kitchen, one stocked with various food items, including two items that could be used to make a salad—lettuce and tomatoes. Over the next couple days, you go to the store and you buy additional ingredients for your salad: cheese, onions, and sunflower seeds. One day, you make the salad. It's delicious, and you have leftover ingredients: the lettuce and the tomatoes. Are those two items now forever considered to be a "part of a salad" (meaning you can *only* use them when you plan to make that specific salad again) or can they be stand-alone, uncategorized food items that simply exist in your kitchen?

You're probably thinking: They would just be stand-alone items . . . You could use the lettuce in a sandwich and the tomatoes in a pasta. Right? Sure. This makes sense.

We don't have this type of mentality or thought process when it comes to our human experiences (especially the ones related to our emotions and behaviors), but we should. Our human experience is far more similar to this salad metaphor than it might seem.

Think about your body, brain, and mind. Each of these parts of yourself has certain ways they function, including ways that could be pathologized under a mental health disorder or condition—such as anxiety, anger, and the desire to escape pain. Over the next few years, you go through life and experience things that cause you to function in additional and new ways: fear of abandonment, trouble regulating emotions and relationships, and perhaps paranoia. One day, you're diagnosed with a mental health disorder that encompasses each of these symptoms. You work to heal yourself, and yet you still find yourself with some of these emotions, feelings, and behaviors. Are these experiences now forever considered to be a "part of your diagnosis" or can they be stand-alone experiences that all humans go through, yourself included? Barring extreme intensity and inappropriateness to the context, of course.

It's easy to separate the ingredients of a salad into their own individual functions. Why? Because it's a fucking salad, it's not really life or death, and it doesn't make a huge impact on most people's lives. It's not so easy to separate the symptoms of a diagnosed mental health disorder from normal human behaviors. Why? Because the trail of hurt and pain the symptoms have likely left are overwhelming, charged, and regrettable.

This is where I found myself that January morning after everything happened with Max. I didn't see myself as a human being. I saw myself as a person with borderline personality disorder who deserved whatever happened to her in life, and a "therapist," "mother," "wife," and "business owner" who had failed and was bound to see more failure in the near future. My brain was helpless, and I was sure my life was telling me I had completely lost control of it. So, I self-sabotaged, but didn't actually do anything that should have led to that decision. I couldn't see that at the time. The grace and space I am so determined to provide my clients I refrained from showing myself. By my own self-imposed criticism, everyone else was allowed to be a human being except for me and I needed to punish myself for my imperfections.

Before you begin your journey, read over this list, and if you experience any of these behaviors along your healing path, don't take it as a

COMPLETELY NORMAL HUMAN BEHAVIORS*

Feeling disconnected from your body	Feeling controlled by your past
Feeling overwhelmed by your body	Feeling the emotions of other people
Experiencing unwanted emotions	Copying other people's behaviors
Not being able to feel desired emotions	Making decisions without knowing why
Engaging in actions that misalign with your words and values	Not knowing what you're feeling
Making assumptions	Getting trapped in negative thought loops
Making mistakes (more than once)	Wanting to avoid pain and seek pleasure
Judging others incorrectly	Feeling not good enough
Thinking you're right when you're wrong	Having difficulty motivating yourself
Thinking you're wrong when you're right	Struggling to accept how things turned out
Not remembering events in your past	Feeling and, at times, being "out of control"

---

* Come back to this list again and again and again. These things are normal. Don't ever let someone tell you otherwise. They can become disordered, yes, but they aren't objectively.

sign that you're failing or should give up or backtrack. Take it as a sign that you're a human being *first* (before all roles and requirements), that your unconscious is showing, and then do something about it.

human first.

The above image is an exact replica of one of my tattoos—my "human first" tattoo. I have several mental health–related tattoos on my body, ranging from a hand carrying a brain around on a string like a balloon, a girl with a mask as her face revealing the darkness behind it, and a skull with a lock across its forehead with a quote that reads "free your mind." However, this tattoo has a very special meaning—one I'd like to share with and offer to you.

"Human first" is the perspective that your, my, their, our, everyone's humanity comes first. It's a phrase that reminds you to consider your own and others' basic human needs, respects, and rights before engaging in any action. It's holding empathy and compassion before judgment and shame, for you and everyone you encounter.

I placed this tattoo on my body to remind myself of the need to be free from demand. Free from conceptualized barriers of my humanity. Open and willing to see an unadulterated reality—one created by myself, not others. As I have with my online audience, I want to offer you the option to get this tattoo placed on your body as a reminder of your own humanity as well.* Community members from my online

---

* I hear they make semipermanent tattoos these days, so hey, less commitment! You will always be a human first, though. Forever.

platforms who have gotten the tattoo have reported feelings such as "I needed this reminder more than I expected," and "It feels like my internal and external are actually matching a bit more. Truly, thank you!"

You may take a stencil directly from this book to any tattoo artist or you can go to my tattoo web page (*thetruthdoctor.com/tattoos*) and choose from five other "human first" tattoo designs we've created. Completely free.

Now, where were we?

Ah, yes, you being in control and choosing what this upcoming 12 Steps of Consciousness journey is going to look like for you personally.

Turn On, Tune In, Drop Out, and Be Here Now

It's 1960, and Harvard has a new recruit. His name? Timothy Leary.

A psychologist known for his unconventional teaching methods and penchant for ruffling feathers, Timothy was about to take Harvard by storm. Little did he know his arrival at the prestigious institution would lead to an encounter that would change the course of his life and that of his new colleague, Richard Alpert.

Richard was already a respected psychologist at Harvard when Timothy joined the faculty. Known for his work in human personality assessment, Richard was the epitome of the traditional "academic"—the prototype, if you will. But the winds of change were blowing.

There was a counterculture movement taking place in American society at the time—a rising culture of peace, love, social justice, and revolution that desired to reject consumerism, celebrate diversity, and experiment with new ways to live. Both Timothy and Richard were drawn to it.

They believed psychedelic substances, like psilocybin (a naturally occurring psychoactive compound found in mushrooms) and LSD, could unlock the hidden realms of human consciousness. So they began a series of groundbreaking psilocybin experiments at Harvard that would become known as the Harvard Psilocybin Project—a project that hypothesized psychedelics could expand consciousness, increase spirituality, and treat depression and anxiety.

Timothy and Richard didn't just sit around casually interpreting their study results. Not only did they roll up their sleeves and directly administer psilocybin to willing participants, including students and colleagues, under controlled and supervised conditions, but they also took the drugs themselves—and not always with the same safety parameters in mind.

In Timothy's archives,[1] photographs and records display long nights that blended into mornings, rooms filled with people of all kinds on various types of "trips," dancing, laughing ecstatically, with broken doors, dog poop on rugs, and writings from Timothy where, for example, he wrote a question mark for his age and listed his current job as "ANGEL."*

Regardless, their actual research results were nothing short of mind-blowing—in the literal sense. Participants reported mystical experiences, the dissolution of their egos, and a sense of profound interconnectedness with the universe. Conventional psychology's rule book fell apart as Timothy and Richard ventured into uncharted territory.†

Their findings didn't just raise eyebrows; they set off a controversy firestorm. Harvard and many other academic establishments were shaken, and society wasn't sure whether to applaud or condemn their psychedelic exploration. Just a few years into their research journeys, both men were fired from Harvard, banished from academia, and discredited for their lack of scientific rigor and adherence to ethical guidelines.[2]

Luckily for them and for us, this was far from the end of Timothy's and Richard's stories and far from the end of their own individual consciousness journeys. Timothy, always the wild one, embraced a more alternative, nonconformist stance. He coined the famous phrase "Turn on, tune in, drop out,"[3] urging people to explore altered states of consciousness and ditch societal conventions. He became an icon, a counterculture celebrity, advocating for the widespread use of psychedelics as a tool to reach a societal shift in consciousness.

Richard's journey took a different turn. Disappointed that their psychedelic research didn't solve his spiritual questions, he traveled to

---

* These were either incredible journeys or scary fucking experiences—probably both.

† It was becoming increasingly evident that psychedelics could be a key to unlocking deep insights into the human psyche, and people were tripping out about it.

India, had a transformative encounter with a spiritual teacher, adopted the name "Ram Dass,"[4] and began his exploration into consciousness through self-discovery. He emerged as a prominent figure in the world of spirituality, bridging Eastern philosophy with Western psychology and advocating for a more mindful and heart-centered approach to life and to consciousness. His book *Be Here Now*—a 416-page consciousness manual encompassing spirituality, yoga, and meditation—became a popular guide for the New Age movement (and the wallpaper in the lobby of the first mental health and addiction treatment center I founded in 2017).

Both men were pioneers of conscious exploration of the unconscious in their own respects.[5] Each of them made a personal choice when it came to how they wanted their journey to look, feel, and play out. Just as they followed their unique paths, you can and should, too. The choice is yours. **You are in control.**

Your 12 Steps of Consciousness Journey

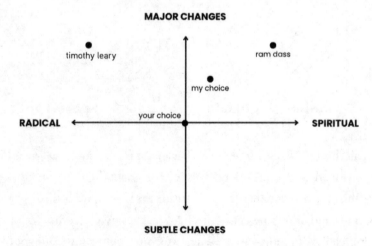

I've left significant room for you to curate your journey based on your individual preferences, needs, wants, and strengths. Remember, only you know what you can and want to experience. You decide how radical or spiritual, major or subtle you want the journey of controlling your life to be. *Your consciousness, your control, is all your own.*

Timothy's saying, "Turn on, tune in, drop out," and Ram Dass's phrase, "Be here now," contain four actions to keep in mind along your 12 Step journey—let's call them "T.T.D.B." for short.

Turn on: Turn on your flashlight—explore your unconscious. (This is required. You aren't going to move forward if you don't see what's holding you back.)

Tune in: Tune in to what's happening; look at your external inputs and the material things around you. Your unconscious is constantly paying attention. You should be, too. There's a reason mindfulness is such a powerful tool. It's you taking control back over your perception, taking it from your unconscious and giving it to your consciousness.

Drop out: Drop out of what's not working. Stop the patterns. You're literally the only one who can. Commit to change, to choice, **to being in control.**[6]

Be here now: Whenever meaningful, be in the moment. Consciousness lies within.

T.T.D.B.

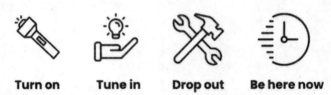

Turn on   **Tune in**   **Drop out**   **Be here now**

If all this feels like a lot to do, it's because it is a lot. Your feeling is likely proportionate and appropriate. This is hard work. If you had no idea you were this out of your own control (read: that you have a three-part unconscious and are 95 percent out of control at any given moment), then it's not really your fault you are where you are when it comes to your level of consciousness. And, now that you do know, you need to do something about it.

This is your opportunity to normalize your own pursuit of consciousness. You're here now. The more you do the work, and the more you destigmatize and embrace this endeavor, the more you encourage those around you to embark on their own unique journeys of self-discovery—and I know you know someone around you who could use some "light work," if you know what I mean.

The Generational Unconscious

I recently read Helen E. Buckley's poem, "The Little Boy." The poem is said to be about creativity and innovation. But I see something else, something deeper, and wonder if you will, too.

The story centers on a little boy who starts school excited to express his creativity, to learn about himself, and to be his own person. When he's told his class is going to be drawing during art time, he eagerly gets his crayons ready and starts thinking about what he's going to draw. (He really likes cars.)

But before he can begin, the teacher instructs all the students to wait. They all need to be ready at the same time. The students are then told to draw flowers, nothing else. The boy dulls in energy but listens and begins drawing with blue and orange crayons. However, the teacher stops him to demonstrate how to make a flower the "right" way, *red with a green stem*, like her and his fellow students.

Despite liking his own flower more, the boy conforms and replicates the teacher's example, *red with a green stem*.

This pattern continues with a clay project. Eager to make dishes of various shapes and sizes (thin, square, tall), he is again told to wait and then to follow the teacher's example of a deep dish, nothing else.

It happens again and again. Over time, the boy stops creating original designs, stops imagining what could be, and only makes what he is shown. Pretty soon he doesn't make things of his own anymore.

After moving to a new school, the boy sits down in class and waits for instruction. However, this time, the teacher encourages him to create whatever he wishes in any color he'd like. The little boy doesn't understand. He doesn't have thoughts of his own anymore.

Sitting at his desk alone, he starts making a picture of a flower, and it's *red with a green stem*.

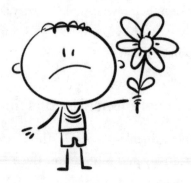

When I read this poem, I see the relationship between what's happening to the boy when it comes to his creativity, his ability to innovate, and how the teacher is limiting his experiences, and I see the *bigger* picture.

From the moment we are born, we are surrounded by teachers—not just in the classroom. Our teachers are our societal guidelines and rules, the concepts both unknown and cherished within our cultures and languages, the beliefs and perspectives of our caregivers and community members, our peer, academic, and vocational environments, and the lessons we teach ourselves as we go through life.

Before we know it (from the moment we're born; so, literally *before we are capable* of actually knowing it), we are instructed toward an inauthentic, curated-by-others identity and idea of what it means to be a human being. An adulterated reality before we've become adults. While acculturation and/or assimilation into one's environment is often necessary for survival, it tends to go to the extreme in many cases—especially when the environment or caregivers lack the understanding of what exactly they're molding: that is, the preciousness that lies in each individual human being as their own individual entity.

The title of an opinion piece in the *New York Times* from February 2022 read "If Everything is 'Trauma,' is Anything?"[7] and I couldn't agree more. As a licensed clinician, I understand the importance of allowing you to decide what has been and has not been traumatic in your life. As I mentioned in the beginning of this book, therapists know they're not in control (of anything when it comes to your life). And the article posed a valid point.

While, as Nick Haslam from the University of Melbourne notes,[8] embracing of the word "trauma" leads us to better understanding the effects of physical and mental harm, over time, the word "trauma" has also lost precision. Thinking back to Chapter Five and our psychoanalytic unconscious desire to make concepts so we can understand our world, it's sort of like our IKEA concept room of "trauma" now holds absolutely everything that's ever harmed us or changed us in a negative way, and it's getting confusing to sort through—for some, individually, and overall, collectively.

It's important to admit that most of the world is completely unaware of how to truly care for the conscious human beings that live in it. Yes, we experience trauma. A lot of it. And we have what's known as **generational trauma**—the transfer of historical and collective trauma from one generation to another. There are two main types of life experiences that fall under the category of generational trauma: society- and culture-based experiences (like wars and discrimination) and personal, familial experiences, like abuse, neglect, and violence. These things are real, and significantly (at times horrifically) damaging.

And, what about the individuals who have been significantly affected by their external environments yet do not fall under one of these categories? There's a better term to use to describe the transfer of one person's or a group of people's unconscious onto another's. Perhaps not *everyone* has generational *trauma*. "Trauma" is a specific type of stress—it's "traumatic stress." Perhaps everyone has, instead, a generational *unconscious*.

The **generational unconscious** is a term I've created to describe the transfer of historical and collective unconscious behaviors, emotions, feelings, and judgments from one generation to another. It describes how the three parts of your unconscious are affected by the life experiences of yourself and your ancestors. Without having to box everything into "trauma," we can begin to tell ourselves a more truthful, non-pathological story of why we are the way we are. Sure, many of the things we've done as humans are clearly pathological, and, overall, we as a species are not. We're just lost, unaware of our unconscious, pretending like we're in control when, most of the time, we're really not.

If you were raised in an environment that knew nothing about what you read in Part I of this book, you likely weren't taught how you functioned as a human until now, or until you took the time to learn about how humans worked on your own. Every day you were unaware, your unconscious gained more power and absorbed more unfiltered information. Yes, it learned ways to help you survive, but you didn't need *all* the ways your unconscious helped you up until this point (especially not the ways that make you feel miserable or hate yourself). And you certainly didn't need everyone else telling you, showing you, and making *you* adjust to *their* own unconscious desires.

You needed a conscious upbringing. You needed conscious relationships. You needed a conscious community. You needed your consciousness cared for.

Now, trauma is important to address. It's real. I know this both personally and professionally. But, here's the real underlying problem: We cause others and ourselves trauma when we don't acknowledge, accept, and work with the fact that we are unconscious beings, naturally, innately, intentionally. We're meant to be unconscious, *and* we're meant to understand that we are and to harness our consciousness, to ensure our unconscious is put to good use. Just because we're meant to be mostly unconscious doesn't mean we can allow ourselves to run automatically in ways that harm ourselves, others, and the world. It's unacceptable if we have any hope for a more unified, conscious, human-focused future.

Fundamentally, it is the lack of conscious awareness in both ourselves and society that has been the largest catalyst of human suffering throughout all of history. It's a bold statement, and it's the thing I believe to be most true in life. My *truest of truths*, as the Truth Doctor.

GENERATIONAL UNCONSCIOUS

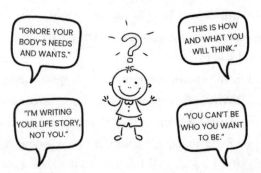

So, what does the generational unconscious look like, how can you spot it in your own life, and what can you do about it? The generational unconscious shows up in each of the three parts of your unconscious—somatic, cognitive, and psychoanalytic.

Let's start by discussing how it shows up somatically.

Your **generational somatic unconscious** is the transfer of historical and collective body-based behaviors from one generation to another. Where the somatic experiences of your caregivers—their responses to pain, their attitudes toward health, their eating habits, and even their unspoken emotional reactions—lay down patterns that you, often unknowingly, follow.

Consider a parent who consistently complains about being in pain yet doesn't go to the doctor or change their lifestyle choices. Physical reactions and ailments often go unaddressed in families, dismissed as inconveniences rather than signals of the body requiring attention. Such behavior, observed by children, becomes a template: Be quiet about your pain or ignore it until it consumes you.

Dietary habits are also silently transmitted from one generation to the next. Overly strict or completely unregulated approaches to food, rooted in how your caregivers ate, shaped your relationship with nourishment. For example, being forced to finish a plate of food regardless of hunger, or being shamed for certain food choices, teaches compliance to others' expectations rather than listening to your own needs.

Body image, too, is not immune. The relentless barrage of idealized body types from media, coupled with what the people around you think about certain bodies, can often instill a deep dissatisfaction and a desire to conform to external standards, at the expense of personal acceptance and self-esteem.

Emotional expressiveness, or the lack thereof, is another trait that we inherit, for good or bad. Children learn to interpret emotions not just from what is said, but from the nonverbal cues that parents unknowingly exhibit. A parent who consistently presents a façade of calm while displaying signs of distress sends mixed signals, making you doubt if your read on how someone's feeling is accurate (making it easier for you to be manipulated or wrong).

It's blatantly clear: When those around you are unaware of how their own bodies function and deserve to be treated, they tend not to treat (or teach you how you treat) your own body with appropriate levels of care.

Now, the thought-based beliefs, biases, and behaviors that are passed down your family, affecting everything from your worldview to your interpersonal dynamics, is the **generational cognitive unconscious**.

From a young age, you were taught to navigate life within the confines of your inherited belief systems. For instance, your parent demands you marry "rich" or that you don't date a "foreigner" or tells you that men are useless or that a woman's place is only in the kitchen. It happened since you were a child, and now you're afraid to veer away from what they taught you, even if you don't know it. These teachings instill a fear of deviating from such expectations, making you only think what society and others want you to think.

Your choices became limited based on allowable perspectives and who the decisions would impact (yourself, others, or the collective). For example, maybe you were only allowed to engage in activities the whole family wanted to do or else it was "selfish," or a different sibling was always given priority or you were told you think "too slow." Eventually, you learned to look to others to make your decisions and you don't give yourself enough time to decide what you really like, want, or need.

Ego-based righteousness further complicates our ability to interact authentically with the world around us. Being raised in an environment where authority figures claim infallibility, as in the saying "I'm always right because I'm the parent," may make you believe that power justifies correctness. "I have the power, therefore I should control you." It doesn't. In fact, this mindset hinders our capacity to appreciate diverse perspectives and to understand that authority does not automatically equate to *truth*.

And lastly, the **generational psychoanalytic unconscious**. This refers to the deep-seated psychological patterns that are passed down, sort of like Jung's collective unconscious. You have conceptual limitations, meaning there are bounds to your mindset created by your environment and the perspectives of those around you. For example, perhaps your family defined "success" through an Ivy League education and marrying into an elite family lineage, or maybe "respect for others" meant abiding strictly to their rules and not having your own opinion. These limitations led your mind to be filled with thoughts of failure and being a bad person because you aren't living up to others' conceptual and prototypical ideals. Growing up under these pressures can create feelings of inadequacy when you fail to meet such standards.

Moreover, your attitudes toward pleasure and responsibility have been influenced by your early environment. For many, due to circumstances growing up, we witnessed dangerous levels of substance use, gambling, and other types of pleasurable behaviors as routine in our daily lives. Exposure to excessive indulgence or risky behaviors as coping mechanisms for socioeconomic stress become hard-to-break habits, even in changed circumstances. Now, although we may live in opposite circumstances, we still feel most comfortable in unsafe situations with potentially unsafe people. The normalization of seeking comfort in harmful ways makes sense when it's all you've ever known.

Additionally, witnessing caregivers or communities struggle without the means to improve their situation instills a sense of lack of control from a young age. For example, perhaps you witnessed your parents struggle to make ends meet, even with multiple jobs, or you watched your aunt's health decline with no cure for her fatal illness even though she tried her hardest to survive, or maybe your hometown was destroyed by a natural disaster in your youth. This ingrained helplessness, held by a perceived global lack of control, often carries over into adulthood, making it difficult to feel in control or capable of overcoming challenges. It's easier to fall into feeling helpless when things go wrong these days than it is to feel like you have the ability to control what's coming next. You're not alone in that feeling.

We live in an unconscious and conscious world with unconscious and conscious people as unconscious and conscious beings ourselves. That's a recipe for a messy human existence. We have a lot of cleaning up to do, but for now, let's focus on you. It's time to sort through all the parts of you that have been curated by others. It's time to get more self-conscious than you've ever been before.

Let's Make Being "Self-Conscious" a Good Thing

In the book *The Body Keeps the Score,*[9] Bessel van der Kolk, a renowned trauma researcher, suggests that people typically experience positive outcomes when they *consciously* establish a connection between past traumas and their present situations. He emphasizes that the first step toward healing is to sense, name, and identify the internal processes and emotions at play. In other words, people feel better when they see how what's "not there" impacts what "is." The first step to healing is to see and name the experience.

This is important. While van der Kolk is referencing trauma, we can again expand this to look at the whole unconscious experience we have as humans. The process by which someone connects a past trauma to their present situation is exactly the same process as when someone connects their unconscious to their consciousness. We're just using the overall human condition versus the conditions of a specific event or series of events. Your unconscious uses your past to make its decisions, and your consciousness lives in the present moment, in the "now." When you establish a connection between them, positive outcomes and healing happen.

So, then, why does being conscious of certain parts of ourselves feel so bad so often?

It makes sense it feels bad to look back at and analyze trauma you've experienced in your life—by definition, trauma is something significantly distressing and disturbing, at minimum. It makes less sense why so many of us feel so much pain when looking at ourselves on a fundamental level in general.

I've come to the conclusion that the very act of being "self-conscious" has been stolen from us. The act of looking at ourselves is presented in many of our lives as something we should and must do when we mess up, when someone doesn't like something about us, or when we aren't fitting the mold of what's societally expected.

If you were given a metaphorical flashlight to look inward on the first day you were born, it's as though the world instantly handed you one with a predeveloped filter, just to show you where you're not fitting in.

SELF-CONSCIOUSNESS

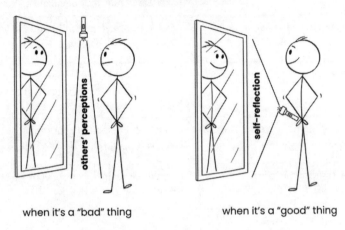

when it's a "bad" thing   when it's a "good" thing

Think about it.

Have you ever really looked at yourself unfiltered? Meaning nonconceptually, nonjudgmentally, without rejection of the physical sensations that arise while you do so. I haven't. I've tried, and I'm getting there, but I'm not there yet. I bagged on monks' lifestyles in Part I, so let me balance that out here by saying I think they've mastered this ability—the ability to see oneself outside of human mind–based conceptualization. I hope one day both you and I can experience such selfless observation of ourselves. I trust that we will, especially as we remain willing to work toward it.

Until then, here are some rules to follow while taking back the power of and engaging in the act of being self-conscious throughout the 12 Steps.

RULES FOR BEING SELF-CONSCIOUS

Dos	Don'ts
Do accept feedback.	Don't let the feedback be the only thing you eat to fuel your decision-making.
Do embrace self-reflection.	Don't look at yourself through the lens someone else gives you. Fuck that.
Do practice self-consciousness.	Don't only practice it when you feel "bad." "Good" things require attention, too.
Do challenge negative self-talk.	Don't let it dominate your thoughts. You're in control.
Do learn from mistakes.	Don't fear failure. Control your response to it.

Fierce self-consciousness requires fierce self-compassion.[10] As you turn the page to begin Step 1, find a way to not forget this—write it down, make it your phone wallpaper, do something to remind yourself that this journey is yours, you control it, you want it, and you *are* self-conscious because . . . you should be. We all should be. It's our human right.

Here we go!

CHAPTER 6 SUMMARY

- You're a human first, before all else.
- You are in control of what your healing journey looks like.
- You may not be to blame for your life, but it's your responsibility to change it.
- Not everyone has generational trauma. Everyone has a generational unconscious.
- You deserve to be self-conscious. It's your right.

7

See Yourself

Self-Awareness and Self-Acceptance,
Steps 1, 2, 3, and 4

In 1993 a short poem was written about someone's life falling apart repeatedly (and avoidably) before they finally did something about it—incrementally and successfully. The poem is Portia Nelson's "Autobiography in Five Short Chapters."[1] It's one I wish I had read anytime between when it was released and when I *actually* ended up reading it—twenty-six years later, in 2019, after I had somehow allowed my life to almost fall apart all over again.

Her words paint a simple yet powerful depiction of the 12 Step journey you're about to begin—the same journey I had to venture through to write this book for you.

The poem tracks a woman's learning curve with a repeating problem: a hole in the sidewalk. Upon her first walk down the sidewalk, she falls into the hole, yelling "I am lost. I am helpless. . . . It is not my fault!" She struggles to climb out.

The next few times, she spots the hole but still falls in, either out of denial or habit, and continues to refuse responsibility. Gradually, she begins to recognize the hole and her habitual mistake, admitting she's part of the problem and quickly getting out. Eventually, she smartens up, walking around the hole entirely. By the end, she's had enough and makes the seemingly simple decision to go down a different street with a different sidewalk.

We've all been there: walking down our metaphorical street of life, falling into the same metaphorical hole over and over again. Whether the street holes in your life manifest as you completely ignoring the needs of your body, acting on thoughts you wish you could ignore, or self-sabotaging psychological tendencies, your unconscious is the one digging the holes and pushing you in.

The accepted definition of insanity, in a court of law, has nothing to do with mental illness. Insane people are not "severely mentally disordered people" as many seem to think they are. Instead, insanity is "unsoundness of mind." It's lacking an understanding that what you're doing or did or planned to do was wrong, irrational, illogical . . . harmful—like repeatedly falling into the same hole on the same sidewalk and saying it's not your fault.

How many people do you know that you'd give this conceptual label of "insane" to? How many people do you know who do the same thing over and over again hoping things will change? They buy the gym memberships, but stop going after three weeks. They put the drink down just to pick it up again. They say sorry and act worse the next time around. They are the ones you know want to be better, but can't seem to make it stick.

I know so many of them.

And I am one of them.

As I've said, we all, *every human*, have work to do if not in our life overall, then at minimum in a few areas important to us—like reducing how often we judge others or learning how to stop caring for ourselves so inconsistently. While we're not going to go to jail for those types of insane behaviors, we often place ourselves in our own personal prisons when we don't address and change them.

Much like Portia's encounter with the hole in the sidewalk, learning about your three-part unconscious and how it's been pushing you into the dark holes in your life may result in surprise, confusion, and even denial. The line "I am lost . . . I am hopeless" that comes after the first time she falls into the hole very much describes how I felt when I first realized the pervasive influence of my own unconscious patterns.

The statement "it isn't my fault" that comes right after was my perspective at the beginning of my journey, too—I wasn't ready to take accountability for the first nine months after my family's January incident and to be honest, not really for the first twenty-nine years of my life. It was too upsetting realizing how much control I'd let my unconscious have over my decisions—even just for a night. The simple (yet excruciatingly difficult) recognition of being in the grip of unconscious behaviors, without initially understanding their origin or knowing how to overcome them, is where we all begin.

You are here now.

You've arrived at the place where you start making conscious change. You don't have to know what you're doing just yet. The steps are here to guide you.

Step 1: Admit It

**STEP 1—Admit it: Your unconscious is showing and
it's controlling your life.**

When Albert Wu was a hospital house officer (in his first two years of medical residency), another resident failed to notice fluid buildup in the heart of one of their patients.[2] The patient was rushed to the operating room later that night. Word of the error traveled fast; the case was tried before a jury of the resident's peers, with the resident ultimately being deemed too incompetent to be a physician.

This worried Albert. Could he have made the same mistake? Would he have received the same lack of sympathy? Seeing the repercussions of someone admitting their faults, admitting what they unconsciously did or consciously missed, was scary. Often, there is no room for mistakes in medicine. When a physician admits their errors, they risk serious lawsuits, the loss or suspension of their licensure, and responsibility for the loss of human life.

The good thing for you? It's unlikely you're making catastrophic, life-

or-death decisions daily, and instead of being a doctor reviewing a case you've messed up on *in front of everyone*, in Step 1 you're simply being asked to review your life and your decisions *in private* (for now).

Much easier, phew!

However, the fact that you aren't a resident doctor who almost took the life of one of your patients doesn't necessarily make it easier to admit that most of your behaviors, decisions, and reactions are controlled by your unconscious. As much as our brains like to feed us thoughts about how much better we need or want to be as humans, we still don't like to admit it to ourselves.

Looking at ourselves critically has felt like a bad thing for so long that it's only natural to have levels of guilt and shame arise. You've been out of control, and it sucks to realize it. But remember: You are not the only one with a powerful unconscious or the only one facing this battle. Being unconscious is synonymous with being human.

In **Step 1—Admit It**, you'll be asked to acknowledge that a significant portion of your behaviors come from places within you that aren't immediately apparent. You will review and accept that what you read in Part I of this book is true: that you have an unconscious, and that it's blatantly showing to others and to you. You'll identify some of your unconscious patterns over the last year and reflect on situations you engaged in without thinking and without your best judgment. Decisions and behaviors that lead to unintended consequences. Things you want to change and control.

You'll create two lists: one containing unconscious decisions and behaviors and another listing their consequences. The first list will be your *Unconscious List*—a personal and private list of how your unconscious shows up in your life. One for you to sit with for some time. Your list should include behaviors that you look at and say, "Why am I like this?" "Why do I do this?" and "I swear I didn't mean for this to happen."*

---

* If it sounds scary to write down the "bad" things you've done, you're feeling an appropriate emotion. Remember: Courage requires fear.

The second will be your *Consequences List*—the list of what happened when you let your unconscious control your life for the last twelve months. You'll base your *Consequences List* on your *Unconscious List*.

As you prepare to begin Step 1, I have one additional recommendation: Try not to complete these steps alone. Research shows that having an "accountability partner"—someone who will either complete this journey alongside you or who can support you along your own by checking in with you at regular intervals—leads to better outcomes and increased success between 65 percent and 95 percent.[3] Think of someone supportive in your life, go to them, call them, text them, and tell them something like, "I'm about to start the 12 Steps of Consciousness! It's going to allow me to have more control over my life. I'm excited, scared, and wanted to let you know." If you're wanting to begin your journey solo, that works, too. Many healing journeys start in private. We'll revisit working with others in later steps.

For now, all you're being asked to do is take things *one step at a time*. And for Step 1, just one question at a time. Grab a journal and turn your flashlight on; it's time to peek into the darkness.

STEP 1 QUESTIONS

Answer these slowly, respect the process, and keep all your work. It's important.

1. **What have you done to try to make better choices in the past? What was the outcome?** Think actions like learning about psychology and human behavior, going to therapy, using coping skills, reducing substance use, or changing environments.
2. **How much do you understand, connect with, and trust your body?** Why is it this much and not more or less?
3. **Do you relate more to being a cognitive miser, naive scientist, or motivated tactician, and why?** Review Chapter Four if needed.

4. **How in control do you feel of your "life story" right now?** Think conceptually—why do you think and feel the way you do about certain people, places, and things like "family," "work," and "love"?

5. **What was it in your life that led you to pick up this book and start working on yourself?** What is just "unacceptable" to you at this point in your life?

6. **When you look back on the past year, which unconscious choices or decisions did you make that you wish you didn't?** Your answer to this question will become your *Unconscious List*.*

Here's one of my *Unconscious Lists*:

UNCONSCIOUS DECISIONS/BEHAVIORS THIS PAST YEAR

- Ignoring my body's need for food and water every single day
- Frequently correcting Max's actions (when a change would be inconsequential)
- Judging strangers by assuming I know their motivations
- Feeling overwhelmed by outside noise and getting more emotional than I want to
- Numbing my stress with habits that make me feel worse
- Feeling helpless after certain life events didn't go how I expected

---

7. **What are the consequences of these behaviors and decisions?** Think about how they've affected your self-image, physical health, relationships, work/school life, community support, etc. This is your *Consequences List*.

---

* This can be a tough first experience. Take your time. Think it through. May this first list give you the feeling of finally "getting it out."

Here's the *Consequences List* I made using my *Unconscious List*:

CONSEQUENCES FROM MY UNCONSCIOUS THIS PAST YEAR

- Unconscious Choice: Ignoring my body's need for food and water
  - » Consequence: Poor physical health and reduced energy when I want to play with my kids
- Unconscious Choice: Frequently correcting Max's actions
  - » Consequence: A stressed-out husband and a guilty conscience
- Unconscious Choice: Judging strangers by assuming I know their motivations
  - » Consequence: Fewer friends and more isolation
- Unconscious Choice: Feeling overwhelmed by outside noise and getting more emotional than I want to
  - » Consequence: A strengthened dissociative relationship with my body
- Unconscious Choice: Numbing my stress with habits that make me feel worse
  - » Consequence: Delays in project completions and negative self-talk
- Unconscious Choice: Feeling helpless after certain life events didn't go how I expected
  - » Consequence: Addictive physiological habits like procrastination and overwhelm

---

You have now completed Step 1. Bravo! Take your two lists and allow yourself to sit with them. See how admitting to these parts of yourself causes you to change how you think, feel, and behave. It might not feel good. But, it likely already didn't.

You're becoming more conscious of the sensations, thoughts, feelings, behaviors, and decisions you experience and engage in daily—this is hard work manifesting into reality. Maybe now you catch your somatic unconscious saying, "Water would be good right now," and instead of ignoring it, you actually get yourself a glass. Perhaps you've toned down how much you're giving feedback and commenting on someone else's actions. Maybe you've started saying "no" more. Whatever the change is, consciously acknowledge it. You're allowed to admit the "good" too. Be proud of yourself, and . . . believe in yourself.

Step 2: Believe in Yourself

STEP 2—Believe there's a better, more *conscious* version of "you."

You may have heard of the two varying perspectives on intelligence: the "growth mindset" and the "fixed mindset." These two perspectives originally stemmed from research conducted by Carol Dweck, who found that people view intelligence as either "incremental" or as an "entity,"[4] meaning people can either grow and develop intelligently or . . . not. They can learn new ways to think and behave or, as you've likely heard someone say or have said yourself, "People are the way they are, and there is no changing them." Importantly, these varying views impact how we as humans approach failure and setbacks.

Think intelligence is flexible? Then mistakes are lessons that you can do something about next time. (Ding! Increased internal locus of control.) And if it's fixed? Mistakes feel like personal and permanent faults. ("There was nothing I could do anyway"; external locus of control.)

These different mindsets contribute to us consciously making better choices in the future or not. However, it's not just our conscious selves that benefit; our unconscious changes for the positive, too. A Michigan State University study dug deeper to see if the unconscious brain itself reacted differently based on these two beliefs.[5]

Researchers did a study with two groups of students. One group believed they could improve with effort (growth mindset), while the other group believed their abilities were set and couldn't change (fixed mindset). The students had to do a quick task where they spotted the center letter in a series of five letters; sometimes all the letters were the same and sometimes the middle one was different.

The researchers were interested in how the students' brains reacted when they made mistakes, so they measured the brain's electrical activity. Even though making mistakes was part of the task, the key finding was not how many mistakes the students made, but how their brains dealt with these mistakes. The brains of students with a growth mindset showed stronger positive signals when they made errors, and they tended to do better on future tests. The study suggests that believing you can get better at something doesn't just make you feel more positive—it might actually help your brain work more positively.

What you believe doesn't only have an impact on how much effort you're willing to put in, it also makes less conscious effort required in the future because your unconscious brain is happy, too. Remember counterfactuals? Your brain's best motivation is regret. It's okay to say, "I want to and *can* improve." I'd even argue it's required.

In **Step 2—Believe in Yourself**, you'll be asked to imagine a better, *more conscious* version of yourself. One you're ready and willing to experience. One you can grow into. This step will convince you consciousness can grow over time; that this isn't "*just the way you are.*" You'll ask yourself a series of questions and then go through your first three "experiences." Each experience is an exercise that will help you come into conscious contact with one of the three parts of your unconscious. Good luck!

STEP 2 QUESTIONS

1. **How do *you* define your unconscious parts and your consciousness?** Write your own definition of each concept:

    My Somatic Unconscious is _____
    My Cognitive Unconscious is_____
    My Psychoanalytic Unconscious is _____
    My Consciousness is _____

Here's an example of one of my recent client's definitions *(shared with permission)*:

My Somatic Unconscious: This is my body's mind. It can even control my brain's mind sometimes to get me what I need. I ignore this one a lot.

My Cognitive Unconscious: These are the thoughts that automatically bounce around in my head, and I don't know where they come from. It's the choices and judgments I make "without thinking." It's also what judges people and makes me think things I don't want to.

My Psychoanalytic Unconscious: This is my brain's understanding of my place in the story of my own life and the whole story itself. It's like . . . what I thought my entire unconscious was. These are the concepts that let me understand everything, that make everything make sense to me.

My Consciousness: This is my ability to reflect on my body, my brain, and my mind. It's my control. It's like . . . what makes me a human, I think. It's something I want to grow. It's my power if I use it correctly (with my unconscious).

---

2. **What were your beliefs about the "unconscious" and "consciousness" before reading this book?** This is an important question to allow yourself to create a "before" image in your mind, of a place you don't want to return to.

3. **Is becoming more conscious the only choice you have to improve your life? Why or why not?** Trick question: The answer is yes. Every aspect of self-healing involves consciousness—awareness of the problem. Journal extensively on this.

4. **In general, what does a more conscious life look like to you somatically, cognitively, psychoanalytically, and overall?**

Answers to this question may look something like this:

> **Somatically:** I'd actually care about my body and give it what it needs and stop judging it.
>
> **Cognitively:** I'd pause before I talk to people and check my judgments of others.
>
> **Psychoanalytically:** I would see my patterns and broaden my views on myself and my life.
>
> **Overall:** I'd appreciate myself more and feel less overwhelmed and more in control.

5. Are you willing to align with these statements?
    - Your emotions must be felt—**Y or N**
    - Your body is your friend—**Y or N**
    - You're not always right—**Y or N**
    - You have been conceptually conditioned—**Y or N**
    - You are responsible for your own healing—**Y or N**
    - You can make more conscious choices—**Y or N**

If you find yourself struggling to say Yes to any of these questions, start by exploring why the statement is so hard to accept. Was it (or its opposite) forced upon you in the past? What is the emotional charge attached to the concept within the statement and where did it come from?

6. **What are some of the best conscious moments in your life?** These are moments where you vividly remember making a deliberate choice or being intentionally present for something.
7. **What do you think made it possible for you to be more conscious at these times?** Think about things like your stress level, your environment at the time, your goals in that period of your life, who your partner was (or wasn't), etc.

In the first part of the book, you tried out exercises that made you notice things your body and brain do without you thinking about it—like how you can feel the temperature inside your nose or how you automatically answer a simple math problem. These were pretty straightforward tasks.

Now it's time to look at your own life, at the things that have happened to you that are more personal and not as simple as those exercises. The next part of Step 2 is about using active, conscious experiences to send a message to your unconscious that you're in charge and that you're going to work on being more aware and thoughtful starting now.

STEP 2 EXPERIENCES

You have three choices. You may complete all three, one that calls you most, or two that best suit your current needs. I recommend completing all three so you actively assess your whole unconscious.

Visit yourunconsciousisshowing.com/steptwo for a free download-able Step 2 Experiences Template.

1. Body Scan Meditation: Pause. Stay where you are at this very moment (do not adjust or "settle in"). Take a slow breath but keep the position you're

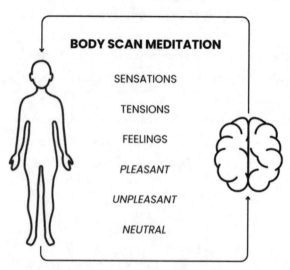

BODY SCAN MEDITATION

SENSATIONS

TENSIONS

FEELINGS

PLEASANT

UNPLEASANT

NEUTRAL

in. Consciously scan your body from head to toe. Notice any sensations, tensions, or feelings in each part of your body. Stay with this for three minutes. Take a long, deep exhale. Now write down or take a mental note of what you intentionally noticed that you didn't notice prior. Because you didn't try to relax too much before the scan, you likely noticed a spectrum of sensory and cognitive experiences—things like how your shoulders were tense, you felt hungry, your feet were warm, and your glasses felt snug. *(Everything you didn't notice before the exercise was controlled and cared for by your unconscious. Your body could feel it. You couldn't. Your brain knew the sensations were happening. You didn't. Wild.)*

The body scan exercise you just completed encourages a meeting between your consciousness and your somatic unconscious. It helps you connect to and therefore gain control over your sensations and reactions. This exercise is now a tool and a skill you carry. I encourage you to do it again and again. Visit your body. It wants you to know it, to help it, so badly.

Bonus: Try to sit with an unpleasant sensation you find for longer than you'd like to—like a pressure point, an itch, or a tingle—without shifting or trying to change it. This will help you learn significant self-control. Sitting through an itch until it passes can be helpful prep for sitting through an uncomfortable meeting or dealing with difficult conversations. It trains your mind to handle discomfort without immediately reacting.

This experience can be uncomfortable for some people. An alternative, perhaps more comfortable, exercise is to choose a body sensation from the list in Chapter Three and track it over a few days or a few weeks, for example monitoring your hunger and thirst levels or the times you fall asleep and wake up.

The ultimate goal of this exercise is for you to start to understand and know how your body feels and what it's trying to tell you. Any way you can become more conscious of your body works here.

2. Delayed Emotional Gratification Test: The next time you're experiencing a heightened emotion in reaction to an event or during a conversation, consciously decide to wait for a set amount of time (like ten minutes) before you share your emotional experience with another person or outwardly in general. Mentally note or write down the emotion you are feeling before the delay and after.

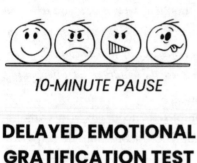

10-MINUTE PAUSE

DELAYED EMOTIONAL GRATIFICATION TEST

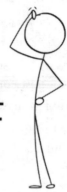

Did the delay change the way you felt about what happened? What was it that changed?

Do you think the delay made you respond to the situation differently?

This is another exercise in self-control. It gives you the opportunity to control both your somatic and cognitive unconscious. In the heat of the moment, good or bad, your body and brain react quickly and emotionally (often resulting in behaviors you don't like). While it's not always practical or the "best move" to hide your emotions, sometimes we need to and we can't. We're impulsive, quick to react. This exercise helps with impulse control. Experience it repeatedly.

Bonus: Do this exercise with opposite emotions—pleasant (like joy and happiness) and unpleasant (like anger and sadness). Log the differences in how you consciously experience each of these delays. Is one type of emotion easier to delay than other? Why?

3. Concept Development Recall: Think back to a nontraumatic (but still emotional) memory from years ago. List the psychoanalytical con-

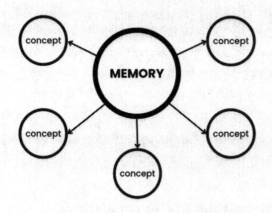

**CONCEPT DEVELOPMENT
RECALL**

cepts related to that memory, and begin to decipher how your definition of each concept played a role in how you experienced the events from that memory.

Here is a nonexhaustive list of concepts to explore as they relate to the memory you choose: *time, beauty, success, morality, fear, happiness, wisdom, good/bad, expensive/cheap, important/not important, attractive/unattractive, moral/immoral, worthy/ unworthy, children, seniors, the "rich," the "poor," "criminals," communication, love, power, authority, etc.*

An example: Let's say the memory is from when someone hit your car in a fender-bender accident and it sent you into a spiral. When you got to work, you were having a hard time staying focused and felt angry at everyone for everything. You spent hours that day being angry. One concept affecting you at the time could have been, well, *time*. You were pissed off because you needed the thirty minutes at work the accident took from you, but then you spent hours mentally damning the person who took less time away from you than you and your unconscious took from yourself by spiraling.

Conceptual tornados of disaster. Stay out of them by asking "What concepts are controlling me right now?" "How else can I see this situation?"

Reflecting on the concepts that live in your mind is a powerful way to tweak the automatic judgments and feelings that come up as you're simply living your life day to day. If you can realize the concept of "time" is what's really causing the biggest issue for you at any given moment, you can redirect yourself and ask "How can I get more time?" (And the answer is usually stopping all the angry rumination your brain is doing and getting your work done instead.)

The conceptual lens through which you view the world determines how you consciously experience it.

Before you move on to the next step, take a moment to appreciate what you're achieving. You're exploring parts of yourself that have always been there but maybe haven't been fully recognized. Many of us struggle with these hidden parts of ourselves, trying hard to be aware and in control, but often feeling overlooked, failing, or just giving up. By doing this work, you're acknowledging your whole self, all the parts, and that's something to feel proud of. Let yourself.

Step 3: Committing to Consciousness

STEP 3—Intentionally commit to consciousness as your tool for change.

On our fourteenth anniversary, giving Max those promise cards at the Big Yellow House Restaurant was honestly the most terrifying choice I've ever faced. The 2012 ultimatum really shook me awake and forced me to start living more intentionally. But this time, I was committed to dive even deeper into this journey of self-awareness, and I chose to do it without my usual way of numbing myself from feeling too much. The thought of truly facing my pain head-on was daunting—I was scared of failing.

Truly committing to consciousness involves some serious reflection on what has to change in your life to make that commitment solid. It might mean altering how you behave or changing something in your environment to keep your mind as sharp and as clear as possible on your path. For instance, I quit drinking for a whole year while I worked through my 12 Steps of Consciousness. On top of that, I also moved our family back to our hometown after eleven years of living in the city where Max and I went to college. I did this to avoid falling back into old, automatic patterns that weren't serving me well. I wasn't going to risk it.

The shifts you need to make might be big or small, depending on what you think you need. If you know you need to make big shifts, go make them. Commitment can only happen when you're ready. Step 3 is about starting a daily practice of consciousness. If you can't commit to the work almost daily, it likely won't work long-term.*

In **Step 3—Committing to Consciousness**, you're making a decision, *the* decision. You're deciding to dedicate your time, energy, and efforts toward using consciousness as the primary guidance tool for your life. You are *committing* to consciousness. This means choosing to pay more attention to how you feel, think before you act, and get to the root of your actions and emotions. Even though this might seem like a quick step in comparison to the others, it's important to think about this commitment for a good amount of time. Allow this step to be a powerful, anchoring experience.

STEP 3 QUESTIONS

1. **What is your greatest fear about being a primarily unconscious human, one that is always, to a degree, "out of control"?** This fear, and the details surrounding it, could be a barrier for your conscious growth. Identifying it and working through it makes success more sustainable.

2. **In what ways have you refused to accept you're not fully in control of your life?** Why has this been difficult for you in the past or present? Why may it be difficult in the future? It's scary to feel out of control, and this fear often makes us want to forget we're unconscious in the first place . . . which makes it worse and strengthens your unconscious tendencies even more. Answering this question gives you insight into potential future barriers.

---

* Daily is not necessary to start off. It may not be required at all. But, if you are blocked, if you are constantly thrown off, triggered, intoxicated, spiraling, you won't have enough control to continue.

This is the first answer I ever wrote down for this question:

"I've felt out of control my whole life. From not deciding to even be alive, to struggling in childhood for basic needs, to experiencing trauma, making huge mistakes, and being told I'm a monster because I can't control my emotions or needs has been really fucking hard. It's just felt like shame. Like I'm the only one who deals with these things. Like my body and brain are the only ones in the world who can't seem to just do life the right way. I refused to acknowledge I was out of control for so long because it was only ever presented to me as a flaw, as a reason to consider myself a terrible person. I worry the guilt and shame and blame and regret will take me out and make me give up in the future."

3. **Are you ready to grow consciously?** What do you need to do to get yourself, your environment, and your life ready for conscious change? What have you not already done?

4. **Are you willing to get uncomfortable (more than you may already be) when you look in your warehouse and see what's inside?** How will you take care of yourself when you ultimately learn something about yourself that's difficult to accept?

5. **What have been the barriers to past commitments you've tried to uphold?** What has made commitments easier to stick with?

6. **Who or what are you completing The 12 Steps of Consciousness for?** Stay on this question until "you" become a reason, if you're not already. We can do things for others, but they don't tend to stick as well as the ones we do for ourselves, too.

7. **What steps are you going to take to remind yourself *every day* you have the ability to make conscious choices?** Step 3's experience is meant to help with this, but you may already have some ideas in mind.

8. **How would your life change if you were to engage in active conscious choices daily?** This is an important one. Allow sequences. "If this, then this, then this . . ."

STEP 3 EXPERIENCE

When your consciousness isn't present, *your unconscious is*. It's making the choices.

Step 3's experience is about helping you consciously remember your ability to be conscious (yes, it sounds a bit silly, but trust me, it's important). When you're not in the habit of paying attention to what's happening inside you and around you, it's easy to get caught up in the hustle and bustle without really living your life. This exercise is designed to help with that.

Visit yourunconsciousisshowing.com/stepthree for a free downloadable Step 3 Experiences Template.

1. Daily Intentional Consciousness: Actively involve consciousness in your daily decision-making. Commit to consciousness daily. Start your day by picking a goal that will guide your actions and reactions. Each morning, for a week or more, spend a moment thinking about how you want to navigate each day's challenges.

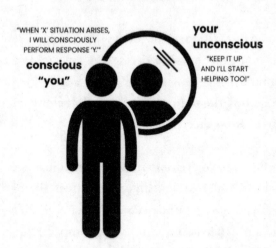

DAILY INTENTIONAL CONSCIOUSNESS

"WHEN 'X' SITUATION ARISES, I WILL CONSCIOUSLY PERFORM RESPONSE 'Y.'"

conscious "you"

your unconscious

"KEEP IT UP AND I'LL START HELPING TOO!"

Phrase it like this: "If this happens, I'll respond like that."

For example, "If my boss is rude to me, I'll stay calm and not react too much." (Though if this is a regular thing, it might be time to consider a new job.) Or, "If I start feeling really emotional, I'll pause for ten minutes before reacting outwardly."

To keep your goal in mind, you can use reminders such as writing it on sticky notes around your space, repeating it to yourself in the mirror before your day begins, or carrying something small like a keychain that brings the intention to mind.

Throughout your day, recall your morning intention, especially when you're about to make a decision. "What is my conscious goal for the day?" This will help you stay mindful and in control. At the end of the day, take some time to reflect on how your intention influenced your choices and feelings.

Bonus: Set a "consciousness alarm" one or two times a day ongoing. Label the alarm "Body, brain, mind," and complete a quick unconscious scan. This could look like asking, "What is my body saying? What is my brain thinking? What is my mind feeling? In this moment." It doesn't need to be more than a sixty-second check-in. This exercise should fulfill the following statement:

"I will check in with my unconscious at [TIME] by [METHOD]." You might set this up as, "I'll check in with myself at twelve p.m. by writing a quick note in my journal."

Extra Bonus: Get the "human first" tattoo so you always remember you're both conscious and unconscious, and how *you* decide how operate as a human. The ultimate commitment![6]

If you're serious about getting the tattoo, visit thetruthdoctor.com /tattoo to download the free tattoo sheet.

With the completion of Step 3, you've *committed* to consciousness. (Yes!) But, here's the catch: In order to actually commit to a life of enlightened consciousness, you have to understand the state of your unconscious, what's in it, and what its intentions (and impact) are, *in detail*. So, while you made the decision to commit in Step 3, in **Step 4—An Unconscious Inventory**, you'll be asked to prove it. For the first time on your 12-Step journey, you'll be asked you to take a deep look at your three-part unconscious, with scrutiny, honesty, and courage.

Step 4: An Unconscious Inventory

STEP 4—Look at the unconscious mess you've been avoiding.

In the 12 Steps of Alcoholics Anonymous, Step 4—where people list their alcohol-fueled behaviors and explore their alcoholic lifestyle—makes many people relapse. It's not easy to admit your shortcomings. And, courage is doing something in the face of fear. If you're not afraid, even a little, then there is no courage. Step 4 in the 12 Steps of Consciousness is a tough step, too, but it's manageable. You'll get through it.

Differently than Step 1, where you reviewed your unconscious decisions and behaviors over the last year, **Step 4—An Unconscious Inventory** asks you to look at your somatic, cognitive, and psychoanalytic unconscious through a series of five different experiences, ranging from connecting with your physical sensations to evaluating the concepts through which you live and judge your life.

You're going to explore the unknown and unseen forces within you with what I call an *Unconscious Inventory*. What do you really value? Which beliefs and concepts are yours and which ones aren't? What does your brain automatically think? What is your body really saying? You'll write all this down, laying it out so you can start to come to terms with it.

You will likely feel defensive and want to stop. It's natural to defend or justify your actions, especially if they don't align with your current, perceived, or ideal self-image. Experiencing multiple perspectives is part of the process. Authentic, conscious introspection requires moving past these unconscious defenses.

You may want it to go perfectly. Why? Because you have a lot on the line. You care about what's been going on in your life, and you want to feel better. Avoid being overly critical—you and your brain have done that enough already.

Think of your *Unconscious Inventory* like looking in and taking a literal inventory of your unconscious. This step is meant to get you to a place where you're telling yourself "Shit cannot stay this way." It's not meant to be comfortable. And you are meant to sit in it.

I am asking you to sit in your shit. And, not only that, but I'm asking you to sit in it *and* not clean anything up yet. (I know, it may make you feel more stressed that you aren't doing anything about it yet. Distress tolerance, my friend, distress tolerance! We will get there. You will get there.)

Your unconscious is going to tell you to look away. It knows where everything is stored already, it has its own organization and prioritization system, and it doesn't want things changing. Ease your unconscious by telling it you're not saying anything needs to go, just that you need to look around and observe. You're sick of your car almost driving itself off a cliff when on autopilot—as you should be.

STEP 4 EXPERIENCES (YOUR UNCONSCIOUS INVENTORY)

The order of the five experiences you'll complete for Step 4 is as follows: (1) Develop your values, (2) look at your unconscious lineage, (3) assess your somatic unconscious, (4) observe your cognitive unconscious, and (5) evaluate your psychoanalytic unconscious. Remember to take breaks and take your time. It may sound or feel like a huge step . . . that's because it is.

Visit yourunconsciousisshowing.com/stepfour for a free downloadable Step 4 Experiences Template.

1. Conscious Values Assessment: Using the Personal Values list below, highlight all the values that resonate most with you and who you want to be. Next, choose only three to five. (If everything is valued, nothing is.) Then, reflect on one to three recent "negative," upsetting life events or decisions that you were in some way responsible for. Analyze how these behaviors and situations relate to your chosen values.

CONSCIOUS VALUES ASSESSMENT

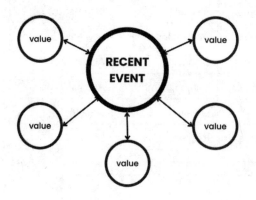

Did they align? Were they at odds? What values did your unconscious focus on instead of the ones you truly desire? *What automatically gets in the way?*

For example, let's say you and your partner get into an argument because you feel hurt, and you decide to call them mean names and criticize their actions. The value chosen by your unconscious could have been "fairness." They hurt you, so you hurt them. But now one of the values you're choosing is "curiosity." Next time, instead of assuming blame and reason, you'll choose to ask questions. "Why did you do this to me?" "What did you mean when you said that?"*

If you're having difficulty determining your values, try thinking about one or two "positive," meaningful memories you have. Looking at the values list, see if you can pinpoint a value you were seeing, experiencing, or feeling in that situation that makes it so meaningful to you. The values you find in each scenario could be the values you find in yourself.

---

* Don't assume. It's usually not a good idea. If you need to, prove yourself right by confirming. Then you'll be double right, always better. (This last part is a joke.)

The goal of this exercise is to show you what your unconscious values versus what "you" value.

28 PERSONAL VALUES
(YOU MAY ALSO CHOOSE YOUR OWN)

Altruism	Connection	Flexibility	Fairness
Dependability	Assertiveness	Open-mindedness	Courage
Integrity	Serenity	Balance	Acceptance
Generosity	Supportiveness	Nonjudgment	Adaptability
Gratitude	Patience	Loyalty	Growth
Well-being	Self-reliance	Responsibility	Stability
Curiosity	Inner harmony	Wisdom	Self/Other-respect

2. Generational Unconscious Analysis: This exercise lets you look at your own generational unconscious—it allows you to see your conditioning and recognize inherited, unconscious beliefs. Take a good look at the behaviors you carry that come from your family, the society around you, and the generation you're part of. Create a list. Think about which behaviors and ideas you've really taken to heart and how they show up in your life. Write them down, getting as detailed as you can. What exactly do these beliefs and behaviors look like when you express them?

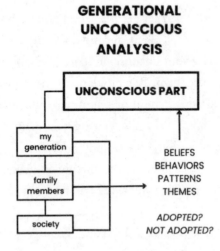

This is not a generational trauma analysis. This is a generational *Unconscious Inventory*. While right now your task is to convince yourself you need to expand your consciousness (which is why we're admitting all the messy unconscious things we've done and had done to us), your unconscious is also very much affected by things outside of the trauma realm, and those should be included as well. Go back to Chapter Six and see which generational unconscious examples make sense. Find which parts of your unconscious are the most conditioned (it may be all of them). Don't shy away from including traumatic details or events if they arise, but don't feel obligated to, either. Sometimes it's too much.

Bonus: Engage in a conversation with a family member about their values and beliefs, and which ones they feel they developed on their own or had passed down to them unconsciously. Note any differences and similarities. This interaction can help you further understand the origin of some of your unconscious patterns.

3. Soma Assessment: This is a two-part experience.

First, assess your relationship with your soma (your body).

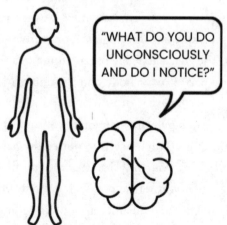

ASSESS YOUR SOMATIC RELATIONSHIP

"WHAT DO YOU DO UNCONSCIOUSLY AND DO I NOTICE?"

Think back to when you felt really in tune with your body, when everything just felt right and balanced—the feeling of a "0" on your Internal Vibe meter. Now, think about the times when you've ignored what your body needs without meaning to or when you've become overwhelmed with its messages. Maybe you've fallen into a morning routine that doesn't help you, like scrolling through your phone for an hour instead of stretching and drinking water. Or maybe you've gotten into the habit of snacking late at night when you're stressed. Remember, you might realize you're doing these things *while* you're doing them, or after, but you don't start out thinking, "Yes, this is exactly what I want to be doing right now, so I'm going to do it." Make a list (yes, another list) of the time periods in your life where you were most disconnected from or overwhelmed by your body. Is there a pattern of people, places, and things that were around?

Where was your consciousness during these times? What were you focused on instead?

RECONNECT WITH YOUR SOMATIC UNCONSCIOUS

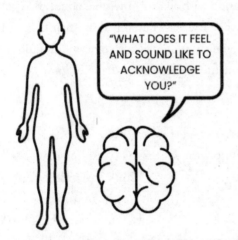

Second, consciously reconnect with your somatic unconscious.

Start by focusing on each part of your body and how it feels, using basic sensations like hot, cold, fast, slow, tight, loose, quiet, loud, strong, and weak as your guide. For instance, get in tune with your hands and arms by trying different activities: Wash your hands, clap softly and then loudly, press your palms together, or gently rub the back and front of your hands. The goal is to really pay attention to and experience each sensation in every part of your body and the automatic reactions of your body systems.*

Doing this helps you close the gap between what you're consciously aware of and your somatic unconscious. You'll begin to notice the patterns, habits, and behaviors that affect your physical health, whether they're helpful or harmful. Like when you refuse to touch your stomach because of the story your psychoanalytic unconscious is telling you. Or when you start doing some of your body parts for this exercise, but then just stop the exercise and move into the next one—the

---

* I can't tell you (I mean, I literally can't tell you) how many clients of mine have cried during this exercise. We're all so disconnected from our bodies. Just clapping our hands mindfully brings tears to our eyes.

one unrelated to your body. (Don't let your unconscious win. It's an easy game to lose.)

Even though this exercise is about getting to know your body better, it might also bring up memories or feelings, some of which might be tough to deal with. That's all part of the process. It's important to fully experience these emotions, recognizing that your body plays a big role in both your joys and sorrows, your strengths and weaknesses.

If the emotions become too much, don't hesitate to look for support. Every *body*'s experience with this exercise will be different, and there's no right or wrong way to feel.

4. Sentence Completion: This activity will shed light on how your mind automatically makes decisions, forms beliefs, and jumps to con-

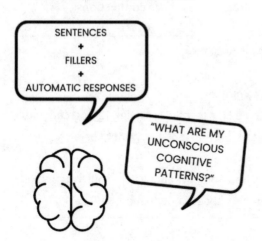

SENTENCE COMPLETION

SENTENCES
+
FILLERS
+
AUTOMATIC RESPONSES

"WHAT ARE MY UNCONSCIOUS COGNITIVE PATTERNS?"

clusions without you even realizing it. Remember "Charlie" from Chapter Four, the part of your brain that tries to take shortcuts? You're going to get a peek at what Charlie is up to— what he thinks, sees, and decides without you consciously knowing, all in the blink of an eye. You'll uncover patterns in your thinking that are guiding how you act.

Complete a list of open-ended sentences with the first and most immediate thought that comes to your mind. Take the sentence structure provided, and fill in the blanks while thinking about different situations, thoughts, or feelings you've had. Once you've finished writing the sentences, look at each one and think about how those thoughts, beliefs, or viewpoints have appeared in your life before, or how they're showing up now. Try to come up with at least one real-life example for each sentence you've completed.

Bonus: After identifying your cognitive patterns, challenge them. For every negative or limiting sentence you've written, counter it with a positive or empowering one.

Here are three different sentence completion templates with filler examples:

I "am afraid of" _____.
Fillers: like, can't, feel, failed, love, regret, am hoping, want to know, etc.
I would feel "happy" if _____.
Fillers: sad, angry, jealous, defeated, surprised, disgusted, etc.
When I am "at work/around my colleagues," I _____.
Fillers: at home, around my partner/s, at my mom's, around strangers, at the end of a line, around people of a different gender, etc.

Here are some of my automatic sentence completions:

Sentence + Filler + Automatic Response

I "am afraid of" being a bad mother.
I would feel "happy" if I could be accepted for being 100 percent me.
When I am "around strangers," I freak out and want to be alone.

Pattern: I unconsciously stress out, on all levels, about what other people may or may not think about or do to me.

CONCEPT EVALUATION EVOLUTION

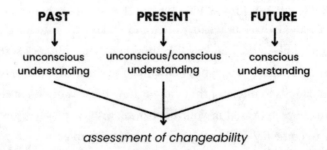

5. Concept Evolution Evaluation: This is the last experience in Step 4. I want you to pick apart various personal concepts that live in your mind. Write them down, along with what you currently think about each of them. Then, try to remember what you would have thought about these same concepts in the past and in the future. Notice how your thoughts have changed over time.

Looking at how your understanding of these concepts has evolved is a great way to see how much you've grown. It's an important part of becoming more conscious. Some of your ideas might be pretty set in stone, while others may have changed a lot. Pay special attention to the ideas that have changed a lot. Think about why those changes happened. Was it a good change or not so much?

Bonus: Engage in a discussion with someone from a different cultural or generational background about these concepts. Compare and reflect on the similarities and differences.

Here's a list of concepts you can start with (add more as needed):

Love	Success	Heartbreak	Failure
Relationships	Health	Education	Work
Family	Leisure	Community	Nature
Adventure	Tradition	Money	Wisdom

Let's say one of the concepts you're examining is "success."

Current definition: Right now, you might define success as having a high-paying job, owning a home, and being recognized in your profession.

Past definition: When you were younger, perhaps success meant getting good grades in school, being popular among your peers, or winning competitions.

Future definition: Looking forward, you might want to define success as being happy with your work–life balance, having meaningful relationships, and contributing positively to your community.

> *Evolution of the definition:* This shows a shift from defining "success" as external achievements and material things to a more holistic view that includes personal satisfaction and helping others.
>
> *Why the shift happened:* This change might have come about due to personal experiences, such as realizing that a high salary doesn't necessarily bring happiness or that meaningful connections are more fulfilling than accolades. Recognizing this shift could be a positive change as it aligns more closely with your deeper values and long-term well-being.

Visit yourunconsciousisshowing.com/stepfour for a free downloadable Step 4 Experiences Template.

POST-STEP 4 QUESTIONS

Complete these questions *after* you have finished the Step 4 experiences.

1. **What do you feel ashamed or guilty about?** You've just completed a massive assignment where you looked into your unconscious and saw how messy it is. It's okay to feel "bad" or overwhelmed or unsettled. Allow it to be there, and sit with these feelings.
2. **Have you always acted primarily unconsciously, or do you feel you've lost or gained control over the years?**
3. **Where did your unconscious come from?** This is one of the big questions. Stay here for a while.
4. **Has anyone hurt you by judging your unconscious behavior? Do you feel anger at this person? Is this anger justified?** These feelings matter. They influence your unconscious decision-making. Explore them.
5. **What feelings do you have the most trouble allowing yourself to feel, and how do you act when you're feeling them?**
6. **Have you ever felt self-righteous** (e.g., certain, *totally* correct, morally superior—like refusing to believe that you could be wrong about

something or someone)? Review situations where your behavior wasn't justified or where you turned out to be wrong. *What's the pattern?*

7. **Do you see any other specific patterns in your unconscious behaviors?** If so, write about them in detail.

8. **Imagine the "worst" parts of your unconscious were placed in the person you love the most.** What would you think of them and their behavior? Would you have any compassion for them and what you know they went through, or would you be mainly critical? What does your answer mean to you? *Explore.*

9. **How do you plan to honor and/or celebrate the completion of your fourth Step?** It's a phenomenal accomplishment. You really should do something!

You've now navigated through the initial, most critical stages of the 12 Steps of Consciousness—Steps 1, 2, 3, and 4. You've admitted your unconscious, started to believe in your consciousness, committed to it, and took inventory of the sneaky ways your three-part unconscious controls your day-to-day life. Venturing through the first four steps might have felt like walking a tightrope at times—challenging, maybe a bit uneasy—but you've managed it with remarkable strength and bravery! Relief comes soon. I promise.

CHAPTER 7 SUMMARY

- You repeat mistakes several times before you fix them because that's how your brain naturally works.
- Admitting you're unconscious is the first step to gaining control—Step 1.
- Believing you can become a more conscious human being is the second—Step 2.
- The third? Actually committing to a life of conscious action—Step 3.
- And fourth? Seeing your unconscious. Looking at yourself (and all your parts) shifts you from autopilot to genuine, intentional self-control—Step 4.

8

Grow Consciously

Admittance, Change, and Amends,
Steps 5, 6, 7, 8, and 9

When you began this book, you encountered a thought-provoking quote from Saint Augustine: "The words printed here are concepts. You must go through the experiences." As you learned in Chapter Five, your entire human reality relies on concepts—the way your brain organizes your understanding of yourself and your world. Each word you've read here, each memory you've thought of, and each sensation you've felt were riddled with concepts. The work and control you feel thus far, however, is a direct result of the experiences you've been willing to go through since Chapter One.

Talk is cheap. You're doing the work. And there's a lot more work to be done.

As well-thought-out as this introductory quote's placement may seem, it goes deeper. How? Well, the story of Augustine's life isn't some irrelevant story about some saint who lived in the fourth century. It's timeless and, more importantly, resoundingly relevant to your 12 Steps of Consciousness journey, especially Steps 5 through 9.

You see, often when we think of historical figures, especially those with "Saint" before their name, we might envision sanctity and purity from birth, from day one. Sort of like how when people imagine a therapist, they often conjure up an image of the prototypical therapist—one in a neutral colored cardigan, over fifty years old, with a bookshelf of subtly colored self-help books and a beige couch for you lie on for an hour—instead of me: someone with multiple visible tattoos, slightly revealing clothing, and a media studio, who wrote a book using the word "fuck" over twenty times. However, just as I've shattered my field's dated expectations, Augustine shattered the typical saint stereotype.

Before becoming the revered "Saint Augustine," he embodied the concept of "rebellion." The tales of his youth and young adulthood could rival any modern tabloid story the media crafts around celebrities and influencers these days.

Augustine was notorious for his hedonistic pursuits—meaning he had many gratification-driven and pleasure-seeking behaviors. (Sounds like the unconscious, don't you think?) He, by self-admission in his book *Confessions* (one of the first autobiographies ever written), led a life filled with indiscretions. His early years were marked by impulsive decisions and an obsession with carnal desires (sex, indulgent sensory stimulations like touch and taste, and more, all rooted in innate human biological, cognitive, and psychological needs). He also had a talent for bending the rules . . . just because he could.

A poignant instance is the seemingly minor act of stealing pears, not out of hunger or necessity, but for the pure thrill of forbidden action. (Ah, youthful fuckery. Those pears were power.) However, getting a little more "toxic,"[1] shall we say: He dated a woman, had a son with her, couldn't and wouldn't commit to her after ten years, refused to marry her (this was huge back in his day), embraced other women (even after he had a *different* arranged marriage—to a child . . .), and admittedly struggled with commitment and impulsive behaviors, something he deeply wished he could change.*

Augustine's behavior also affected those who loved him dearly, including his mother, Monica. Every act of impulsivity, every dive into debauchery, pained her. (I know this feeling. I've seen it in my parents' eyes when they tried to save me from myself, several times.) However,

---

* If this guy can cause this long-winded disaster and still become a saint, I think we can all change.

this wasn't enough to make Augustine change. Well, not for a while, anyway. Years later, amidst the whirlwind of his life, after it all almost completely fell apart, Augustine's trajectory shifted.

Why does it always seem like it has to get to this point? Because we resist what we don't think absolutely *has to* change. It's why in Step 1, your journey started with me asking you to list what thoughts, feelings, perceptions, and behaviors are completely unacceptable to you at this point in your life. Your body, brain, and mind have to *know* it's time to change. You have to give *yourself* the ultimatum.

Like many of us, a series of profound personal revelations prompted Augustine to question his decisions, his values, and his purpose. His internal struggle, and eventual metamorphosis, shine through in his writings, which remain powerful reflections on personal growth and redemption, including the quote I placed at the beginning of this book.

We all have the capacity for profound change. No matter how entrenched our patterns, behaviors, or beliefs, it's never too late to change course. Steps 5, 6, 7, 8, and 9 are all about growing consciously and redeeming yourself in ways you've been needing and wanting to for some time now. You won't become a saint, but as I've said, consciousness doesn't have to be spiritual. The goal for these steps is for you to become more awake, more conscious, more . . . human.

The first step in this chapter is **Step 5—Conscious Honesty**. It's about confession—not in the religious sense but in the raw, unfiltered honesty kind of way. This is the step where you verbalize and share your unconscious patterns, biases, and behaviors with another human being. This may sound scary, and it is scary. As you've learned, and likely already knew about yourself, humans are judgmental, biased, and self-protective. And, at the same time, when we feel safe and secure, we tend to be understanding, curious, and connective. Safety and security come from telling the truth. Think about it; take a second. I'll repeat: Safety and security come from telling the truth.

Sharing the darkness of your unconscious with another person brings accountability to your actions and strengthens your commitment to consciousness even more (it's why I'm so truthful; it's the only thing that's saved me). The process in Step 5 is like stripping down, standing in front of a mirror (when someone else is there), seeing ourselves, and them seeing us . . . fully exposed.

And guess what? It's liberating, and fucking beautiful—no matter what it looks like.

When we put our truths out there, they lose their grip over us. We stop running, stop hiding, and start understanding the reality of what's really going on. I'm so excited for you to experience it.

After showing your unconscious to someone else in Step 5, **Step 6—Prep Yourself** is (you could have guessed it!) a preparation phase, where you're mentally and emotionally getting ready to take action, to consciously change and control your life. This step is the bridge between seeing and understanding your unconscious and actually doing something about it. While you've looked at how your unconscious functions in prior steps, in Step 6 you'll list out specific behaviors that arise from each of your three unconscious parts. It's like taking your car to the shop to be assessed for malfunctioning. You'll look at the body (somatic), the engine (cognitive), and will probably end up asking yourself, "How and where the hell have I been driving lately? Things are pretty messed up!" (psychoanalytic).

Step 7—Conscious Control and Change comes next. During this step, you'll actively engage with the parts of you that need conscious curation—the ones that really need the CEO's oversight, not just their signature. Think of this step as a deep spring cleaning of your unconscious warehouse, ensuring every nook and cranny is addressed, allowing for fresh, invigorating conscious energy and light to flow through. If you don't want to keep falling into metaphorical holes, you need to clear a path that stops leading you there.

In Step 7, you create your *Conscious Growth Action Plan*, one for each unconscious behavior you want to change or control. This is where you will see actionable, real change begin to take place (if you haven't already). You'll come back to Step 7 again and again.

In **Step 8—Unconscious Harms** (arguably one of the most challenging yet rewarding steps, similar to Step 4), you'll confront an essential truth: Your unconscious behaviors might have unintentionally hurt or affected others in ways you wish they didn't. I mean, I'll just say it now to rip the Band-Aid off: They have. You have hurt people when you didn't mean to. It's okay, we all have, even if we're not directly aware of it.

However, instead of just acknowledging this (which doesn't feel very good), Step 8 helps us do something about it. In this step, you make a list of the people you might have harmed, along with the specific instances, big or small, that you can recall. Not just major conflicts that have happened in your life, even subtle ways you might have hurt someone without realizing it (think microaggressions,[2] side comments, and nonverbal reactions you know you made but act like you didn't).

Step 8 is where you begin taking interpersonal responsibility. We beat ourselves up for being human (it's sad, really) and we need to stop (both beating ourselves up for it and allowing it to let us beat up others—literally and metaphorically).

Which brings us to the bold and courageous **Step 9—Acts of Amends**. With humility as your guide, you'll actively seek out opportunities to make right your past wrongs.* To do this, you'll admit your mistakes, make amends, and find ways to make up for what you've done—whether directly toward each person you've hurt or indirectly through community work and actionable lifestyle changes. It's not about saying sorry; it's about understanding the impact of your actions and taking real steps to correct them. It's about healing, reconciling, and developing conscious relationships.

Drawing parallels with Augustine, here's what's evident: Transformation isn't reserved for the saints or the sages. It's a universal human capability—one that can turn you toward sainthood if that is something you so desire. Your journey, much like Augustine's, and Timothy's and

---

* Yes, this an absolutely necessary step. You need to change your world and your environment. You can't grow consciously if you don't relieve your life and those you love from the unconscious pain you caused. Amends are required.

Ram Dass's, and mine, is unique. But the promise of transformation, of rebirth, and of conscious evolution remains constant. It's a journey from who you were to who you can be, and you're on that journey now.

As you complete Steps 5 through 9, remember Augustine's wisdom:

The words here, these steps, are concepts. The real power lies in the experiences.

Step 5: Conscious Honesty

STEP 5—Get honest: Share your unconscious patterns with another human being.

It's time to sit down with another person and get real. In this step, you will share your Step 4 *Unconscious Inventory* and its contents with someone else. (I know, scary! But keep reading.)

Different than the accountability partner you may have chosen at the beginning of this process, this step requires you to seek out someone in your life you can bring into your journey (even if just for this one step). If you'd like the person to be your accountability partner, that works, too. While the first four steps of your journey have been personal, things are about to start getting interpersonal, bringing consciousness not only to yourself but into your relationships.

You're going to embrace vulnerability in Step 5. Ooh, vulnerability. Another word you could say I don't like. Why, you may ask (especially as a therapist)? Well, the *New Oxford Dictionary of English* says vulnerability means "to be exposed to the possibility of being attacked or harmed, either physically or emotionally." And synonyms for vulnerable include "defenseless, frail, weak, helpless, exposed, in danger, and at risk."[3]

Now, the question arises: Who the hell would want to do anything vulnerable when that (hurt, harm, danger) is the potential outcome? I'll tell you who. You and I. Why? Because sharing about our human struggles, our unconscious tendencies, has been tied to "vulnerability" for far too long. We shouldn't be at risk of being attacked or harmed for admitting where we'd like to improve and what's been holding us back. This step is meant to help with that.

Step 5 challenges your fear of judgment and of being vulnerable. It's essential to remember that what you're admitting to are *shared* human flaws—we all have a three-part unconscious that shows, and immense potential for growth. We *all* struggle with being human, and we could all use some time to recover from it.

The success of this step relies on you choosing the right companion (you don't want to have your vulnerability go haywire and get hurt). The right people, the ones who will truly help you progress in life, they see you differently, hear you differently, support you differently. Your humanity, your consciousness, exists to them, even when all they can see is your unconscious. Like how Max and I see each other. How we can "talk about the darkest things we've done, seen, and said in our lives and we can hold them up into the light."

Think about a person who has always treated you like you deserve what everyone else does, even when you didn't think you did. When you're choosing who to share your inventory with, think about how you've been treated in the past, especially when you've behaved unconsciously. There are likely people who've provided you "tough love," those who showed you compassion, those who were right there next to you being just as unconscious, and those who've been the prototype of "a conscious human being" (you know, your friends who act like hippies and modern-day monks). All individuals who have commented on your unconscious decisions and behaviors with different kinds of direction and guidance.

Each of these individuals may help you in Step 5 in different ways. Determine which way would best serve you at this time. Ask yourself: How are you feeling about sharing your *Unconscious Inventory* with another person, and what do you need most, interpersonally, to do it successfully? The goal of Step 5 is recognizing and sharing your "flaws" *without* being consumed by guilt or shame. Be mindful who you choose. You can't undo, erase, or skip this experience. You've already committed to the 12 Steps.

It's okay. **You're in control.** Move forward.

There are two experiences within this step. The first is a self-reflection, the second is when you allow someone else to be your mirror. For some, sitting with yourself for a bit of time (without distractions), allowing yourself to consciously *feel* and *see* your unconscious can be overwhelming. If that sounds like you, you may want to choose showing your unconscious to someone else first. For others, sharing your inventory with another person may be the scariest fucking thing you've ever imagined doing, so sitting with yourself first feels best.

Move forward in the order that makes you most willing to follow through.

STEP 5 QUESTIONS

1. **What is the purpose behind completing the 12 Steps of Consciousness for you?** Use this question as a way to refocus as you begin this new step and new chapter.
2. **How long have you been hiding your unconscious and what you consider to be the "worst" parts of you?** If it feels like you're about to admit "secrets," this process can seem scarier than it needs to be. When reflecting on how long you've felt out of control, don't forget to tell yourself you're gaining control daily.
3. **How do you feel about admitting (and I mean *really* admitting) your unconscious parts to another human?**
4. **Do you believe that completing Step 5 will make your life better?** In what ways? Pump yourself up. Holding all of this in alone isn't what we're meant to do as humans.
5. **Write down the names of the people in your life whom you trust the most and are the most comfortable around.** Do you think one of them would be interested in being your Step 5 companion? When and how do you want to ask them?

STEP 5 EXPERIENCES

There are two experiences within Step 5. The order you complete them in is up to you.

1. Conscious Self-Admission: This experience involves self-reflection. It requires you to look inward, noticing the width of and level of acceptance toward your unconscious *now* compared to when you first finished Step 4. Find time to sit with yourself. Then, answer the following questions:

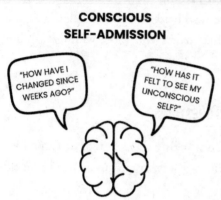

CONSCIOUS
SELF-ADMISSION

"HOW HAVE I CHANGED SINCE WEEKS AGO?"

"HOW HAS IT FELT TO SEE MY UNCONSCIOUS SELF?"

What is your relationship with your unconscious after seeing it? Is it still as scary? As charged? Or are you realizing it's not going anywhere and becoming more comfortable with it? Does it feel controllable?

Let the answers be meaningful. They're so important. Then, choose one or both of the below Conscious Self-Admission exercises.

Meditative Self-Admission: Settle into a comfortable position by sitting or lying down—you want to reduce your body's energy expenditure so you can focus on feeling its sensations and listening to your thoughts. Close your eyes and start to breathe deeply into your stomach (deep breathing not required, but recommended), focusing on the memories and experiences from your Step 4 *Unconscious Inventory. Which revelations were the most profound?*

Maybe it was when you realized the concept of "money" has long fueled your ignorance toward your family's needs. Perhaps it was when you cried because you finally heard your body's messages. Maybe the sentences you completed showed an automatic desire to leave your partner or your job, which you almost knew but couldn't admit. Or it could be you finally realized you live a life outside your true values. Whatever the outcomes were, immerse yourself in them.

Ponder your recent actions and decisions since seeing your unconscious in detail. *Did the impact and meaning of Step 4's experiences come and go faster than you'd have liked?* If so, that's your unconscious showing (and winning) again. (It tends to do that a lot in the beginning. It's okay, keep going.)

This part of the experience is not meant to be a full meditation session. It's meant to have you be as present as possible, with little to no distraction, while you allow all parts of you to reflect. The process can look like: Read a part of your inventory, then close your eyes and reflect, read another, reflect more, and so on.

Mindfulness Self-Admission—Alternatively, if meditation isn't your preferred method, try creating an instrumental, mindfulness-based playlist* and go for a walk in a place you feel comfortable, safe, and secure. You do not have to sit still with your eyes closed to introspect on your inventory.

2. Unconscious Inventory Share: Here comes one of the big interpersonal tasks on your consciousness journey. For this second Step 5 ex-

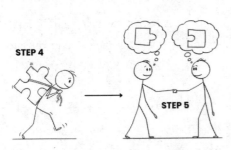

perience, you will take your Step 4 *Unconscious Inventory* and share it with your chosen person. You'll share the insights gained from Step 4's experiences, your answers to Step 4's questions, *and* your reflections on what this all means about you as a human being, as a person trying their best.

Visit yourunconsciousisshowing.com/stepfive for a free downloadable Step 5 Inventory Share Template.

---

* An instrumental, mindfulness-based playlist of songs includes songs with no spoken words that keep you calm and able to still think; you can use mine on Spotify by searching "The Truth Doctor Self-Admission Playlist."

Use this breakdown for your share:

- **Choose Your Companion:** Opt for someone you trust implicitly. This could be a friend, family member, therapist, or mentor. Ensure it's someone who can listen without judgment and keep what you share confidential.
- **Prepare Yourself Physically, Emotionally, and Mentally:** Before the meeting, take some time to reflect on why you're doing this, to feel as balanced as you can. Remember, you're not seeking validation during this process, you're vocalizing your truth and allowing it to be acknowledged by another human.
- **Set the Scene:** Find a quiet, comfortable space where you both can talk undisturbed. Preface the conversation with what you hope to get out of this experience and how important it is for your transformative journey. Also, let your companion know you want honesty in return—this is why you should choose someone whose truth you can handle (both in how they present it and their intention behind it).
- **Speak Your Truth:** Using your *Unconscious Inventory* as a guide, verbally share your admissions. Try to stay factual and refrain from entering a space of self-blame or guilt. Key focus: acknowledgment, not atonement.
- **Listen Actively:** After sharing, allow the other person to speak. They may offer insights, comfort, or share their own experiences. Engage in the conversation, paying attention to the ways your unconscious responds to feedback (body sensations, automatic thoughts, activated concepts).
- **Show Gratitude:** Thank your companion for their time, understanding, and confidentiality. They may thank you as well. Being trusted by someone is meaningful.
  - » **Reflect and Write:** After the meeting, spend some time assessing yourself and how you feel about the experience.

> » How did voicing these admissions turn out?
> » Were there any new realizations?
> » How did the other person's feedback or perspective influence your understanding?

You've now finished Step 5, openly acknowledging who you are and how your unconscious shows. It's crucial to accept your past slip-ups and to be real and true to yourself, admitting both the good and bad parts—even if you worry about being judged. Imagine if we all just said and did things honestly and consciously; we'd all feel a lot less isolated and a lot less like we're the only ones screwing up in life.

Sure, we all have moments of clarity, and many of us experience conscious *moments* in our lives, but the true success of us as human beings will be when we begin to build conscious *lives* and *relationships*—when we can admit to others our flaws instead of doubling down on them just to keep them hidden. When we can tell our truth without getting hurt.

Step 6: Prep Yourself

STEP 6—Prep yourself: Create a list of ways you want to curate your unconscious.

Have you ever seen someone else's "cons" list they made about you?

Let me tell you a story.

In 2010, before the ultimatum and my subsequent BPD diagnosis—so you can only imagine the unconsciousness that was my behavior—I was visiting Max in college (we were on a break) when, upon grabbing something from his closet, I found a black notebook—one hidden where I'm sure no one was supposed to find it.

I opened it. (Of course I did. I didn't understand the concepts of respect or privacy at that time.)

What I saw was a page with my name at the top, a line down the middle, and PROS AND CONS written across the first line. It was a list of all the "good" and "bad" things about me. Admittedly, this was probably a very important task for Max to complete at the time. Like I said, before I was a therapist, I was a bitch.

The details of this pros and cons list have left my memory, but the feeling I had when I first saw the list remains. Was I really so messed up that someone had to write down all the problematic ways I affected their life? Unfortunately, the answer was yes.

This experience was the first time I saw the outcomes of my unconscious behavior listed, literally in bullet points, in front of my eyes. The fact that it was completed by another person was horrifying. And, at the same time, it was as though I was seeing a list of what I already knew was there and was too afraid to admit.

You've learned a lot about your unconscious thus far. However, it's one thing to identify and admit your unconscious patterns and entirely another to be genuinely ready to work on them. Take it from me—when I first saw Max's list of all my faults, I was definitely not ready to deal with them. Hence his need for an ultimatum two years down the line. (If you've noticed, I have an unconscious pattern of not wanting to work on things when it's clear I should.)

While Step 6 is a preparatory phase, its importance cannot be understated. Different than seeing a list of your cons created by someone else and subsequently doing nothing about them, in this step you're being asked to not only create your own list of self-"cons," you're also being asked to understand that you *will* take action on this list moving forward. Tell your unconscious that, right now. And again and again. You *will* take conscious action and **you are in control.**

As I've mentioned many times, your unconscious is not a bad thing. Sometimes it feels good to act unconsciously—like when we just want to be "right" so we decide we are and that's that, or when we decide to engage in and maintain our unconscious habits because they're easier, quicker, take up less energy, and make life simpler for us (or so we think). Habits like waiting until the last minute for things or spending the money you know you don't have. It's called being *human*. We all do it. And, this step is about deciding where in your life your unconscious patterns aren't working, and getting clear about how you're going to change them.

PRE–STEP 6 QUESTIONS

Complete these questions before you complete the Step 6 experience.

1. **What does it mean to you that you can "use consciousness to change and control your unconscious"?** Think about how much being conscious matters to you these days. How has your life changed since Step 1?

2. **How much of this journey is in your control?** Your reflection here will give you insight into where your locus of control currently lies. Revisit the questions from Chapter One for more clarity if needed.

3. **What are the "pros" of your three-part unconscious?** These are important because you aren't getting rid of your unconscious; you're learning to work with it. Think about it like this—when you have to work with a colleague or complete a group project with peers, it's usually much more enjoyable and productive when you like who you have to work with . . . even just a little bit.

4. **Would you say you're an honest human? Have these steps made you more truthful?** Honesty is needed toward others and yourself. If you refuse to admit you're unconscious (especially at times when you're actively engaged in unconscious processes), you may regress and take steps backward (which is also fine; remember: progress, not perfection, my friend).

5. **What are you most worried about when it comes to making *real change*? What can you do to address this worry?** The step after this one is the largest consciousness tasks you'll embark on. Make sure you take this question seriously.

STEP 6 EXPERIENCE

The Step 6 experience is a two-step process.

The first involves creating a list of all the behaviors caused by your three-part unconscious, and the second is you choosing which behaviors you'd like to actively work on—the ones you think will cause the most change in your life, the ones that will give you the most control.

1. Unconscious Change List: Using each of your unconscious parts, create a list of the ways you automatically show up in the world—your *Unconscious Change List.* This list can be as long or as short as you need it to be. Mine was . . . long.

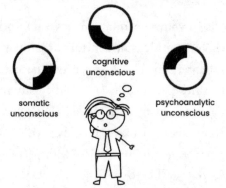

Keep in mind that many of these behaviors will be common. We all primarily function the same way, just to differing degrees. The key to creating your list is to think about if these behaviors present in such a way that it negatively affects you, your life, or others in your life.

Below you will find some of the most common ways our human unconscious shows up. Feel free to choose from this list and also add your own outcomes.

Visit yourunconsciousisshowing.com/stepsix for a free downloadable Step 6 Experience Template.

SOMATIC UNCONSCIOUS

Neglecting Physical Health: Ignoring regular exercise, nutrition, and medical checkups.

Overworking: Pushing through physical and mental exhaustion without rest or relaxation.

Disregarding Pain: Ignoring physical discomfort or chronic pain.

Bodily Tension Reactivity: Frequent bodily tension, such as clenched jaws or tight shoulders.

Physical Harms: Reacting with physical outbursts like hitting objects, others, or self-harm.

Sedentary Lifestyle: Consistently leading a physically inactive life.

Poor Sleep Hygiene: Maintaining irregular sleep patterns and disregarding sleep quality.

Neglecting Real Self-Care: Failing to engage in self-care routines like grooming and hygiene.

Addictive Habits: Substance abuse, overexercise, overeating, or other addictive habits to numb.

Heightened Sensitivity: Increased or decreased sensitivity to personal sensory experiences, and to others' physical pain or discomfort.

Other: _____

COGNITIVE UNCONSCIOUS

Repetitive Thought Patterns: Obsessively dwelling on certain thoughts or worries.

Overgeneralization: Sweeping, negative (or positive) judgments based on limited information.

Automatic Negative Self-Talk: Consistent critical, regretful, or complacent internal dialogue.

Cognitive Misering: Going with the easiest, fastest, most readily available solutions.

Assumptiveness: Believing that what you assume to be true is in fact true, without confirming.

Rigid Thinking: Resisting flexibility in problem-solving, not considering alternatives.

Avoidance of Cognitive Dissonance: Refusing to confront conflicting beliefs or ideas.

Peer Pressure and Mirroring: Engaging in behaviors mainly due to environment and culture.

Anxious: Constantly worrying about potential negative outcomes.

Judgmental: Making snap judgments about people or situations without sufficient information.

Perfectionism: Demonstrating perfectionistic behaviors, such as frequent revising or editing.

Other: _____

PSYCHOANALYTIC UNCONSCIOUS

Avoidance of Self-Reflection: Shying away from introspection and personal growth.

Repetition of Unhealthy Patterns: Engaging in destructive relationships or behaviors.

Secrecy: Secretive behaviors or hiding aspects of one's life, even from close friends or family.

Suppressing Feelings: Consistently repressing or denying feelings rather than processing them.

Self-Sabotage: Behaviors that hinder personal growth or success (may not be repetitive).

Escapist Fantasies: Frequently daydreaming or indulging in fantasies to avoid reality.

Constant Seeking: Constantly seeking out new experiences or relationships to fill a void.

Avoidance: Avoiding or evading difficult emotional situations or conversations.

Fragmented Identity: Struggling to maintain a coherent and stable sense of self.

Other: _____

2. Short List—Unconscious Changes: Next up, you need to condense the big list of things you want to fix about yourself and make it more re-

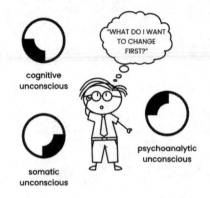

SHORT LIST: UNCONSCIOUS CHANGES

"WHAT DO I WANT TO CHANGE FIRST?"

cognitive unconscious

psychoanalytic unconscious

somatic unconscious

alistic. You've probably spotted a bunch of automatic habits you want to change, but you can't tackle them all at once (no matter how hard you try).

Looking at your *Unconscious Change List*, choose one or two behaviors from each of your unconscious parts you'd like to work on first. (In Step 7, you'll pick behaviors from this short list to start actually changing, so make sure you write down ones you're willing to actually work on.) Oh, and get specific. The more details you give yourself, the better you'll be at noticing the behaviors when they happen.

Example: *Unconscious Change List*—Sedentary Lifestyle: Consistently leading a physically inactive life. *Short List—Unconscious Changes*— Sedentary Lifestyle: Almost always at home, mostly in bed, don't go in the back or front yard, don't walk the neighborhood.

Here's an example of my most recent *Short List—Unconscious Changes*. Notice how I have personalized what each of these behaviors look like.

MY SOMATIC UNCONSCIOUS

- Bodily Tension Reactivity: Constantly tense, feeling tired, jaw getting stuck/clicking, tight muscles, stomach aches, etc.
- Sedentary Lifestyle: Almost always at home, mostly in bed, don't go in the back or front yard, don't walk the neighborhood.

MY COGNITIVE UNCONSCIOUS

- Overgeneralization: Quick to judge most things one way or another (good/bad); fast assumptions get in the way of curiosity and patience (I really need patience).
- Perfectionism: Recognizing too many details and having no coping skills to release attachment to many of them, causing delays and serious anxiety about everything.

MY PSYCHOANALYTIC UNCONSCIOUS

- Decision-Making Struggles: Frequently choosing others' needs over my own and making irrational, more emotional decisions (when they aren't the right ones).
- Avoidant: Refusing to say what needs to be said to people who need to hear it (when it truly goes against my values to do so).

POST-STEP 6 QUESTIONS

Complete these questions *after* you complete the Step 6 experience.

1. **What were your initial reactions to seeing both your extended Unconscious Change List and your Short List?**
2. **What are the thoughts and feelings arising knowing you've prepped this ahead of a lengthy (likely difficult) behavioral change process?** Don't be scared. It's been a long and difficult time already—unknowingly living through the decisions and actions of your unconscious. You wouldn't have picked up this book if it wasn't. What comes next leads to more, not less, control over how you think and feel.
3. **Are you still committed to using consciousness to control and change your life?** You committed to this process a significant time ago. Does it feel like it's getting easier or harder? If needed, how

can you make the process more comfortable? One tip: Try slowing it down. If you've felt rushed or unsettled, perhaps review your past steps. There's no fault in reviewing your work and making changes where needed.

4. **How are you going to celebrate the accomplishment that is completing Step 6?** In Step 4, you listed the ways in which your unconscious works. Now, you've listed what it creates, behaviors that you engage in when you're less conscious and less in control. This is a big deal—you're staring straight at your unconscious. Courageous! Acknowledge that courage. It's how you make it real.

As you prepare to move into Step 7, a step of actionable change, realize you may regress to old, unconscious patterns. Perhaps you already have. Old habits die hard. Slipping backward into old ways doesn't mean failure. It's a part of the process. I'd argue it's not even going backward. It's staying still. But, that's just perspective.

Prepare for the need for patience (and to ask for it from others). Real change takes time. You deserve to celebrate your victories (no matter how small or inconsistent). The journey to becoming a conscious human is an ongoing, slow, forgiving pursuit. But also don't oversimplify this process. It's broken down into steps, and seems simple enough, but some unconscious patterns have deep-seated roots, ones possibly linked to significant past traumas. Such patterns might require professional intervention and can't be simply worked away at lone will. This doesn't mean something is "wrong" with you. It means you need support, like *all* humans do.

Okay, you're prepped, and real, conscious change is coming. You've talked the talk, now let's walk the walk.

Step 7: Conscious Control and Change

Step 7—Do the work: Consciously curate your unconscious.

Over the last seven chapters and six steps, you've explored your three-part unconscious, experienced consciousness, and come to realize the relationship between the two—something I referred to in the beginning of this book as "the only superpower you will ever have."

But what does this superpower actually look like in action? It's not like we're shooting laser beams out of our eyes or slinging webs from our palms. Our superpower lives within us; it's human, not fantastical. If anyone knows this best, it's Batman. Yes, I said Batman.

Did you know that Batman doesn't have traditional superpowers like many other superheroes? Instead, his "powers" come from his exceptional *human* abilities—like control of his body, the ability to decipher his thoughts, and the story he tells himself of his purpose in life. This is mixed with his ability to use tools and techniques really, really well. In Step 7, you'll start living your life like Batman. (Except you'll actually feel your feelings, and won't be such an angry homebody.)

All your parts—conscious and unconscious—are deeply connected, and they all influence one another; a sensation becomes an emotion that becomes a thought that becomes a feeling that becomes a memory that affects how you view future sensations and experiences and so on. *You truly are a universe.*

With that in mind, consciously changing and controlling your behavior involves practical changes targeting several unconscious causes of the behavior itself—things like addressing the automatic physiological patterns of your body, refusing to be manipulated by others, developing strategies to introspect before acting, exercising restraint and patience, adjusting your environment, avoiding emotional activation, and more. You have to make the conscious decision not to fall back into the same holes over and over again, and you have to grow your toolbox of techniques to fight off all the ways your unconscious wants to make you function.

Step 7 is where you put your superpower to work, where you not only see your unconscious showing, but begin to control it by creating and executing a plan I call your *Conscious Growth Action Plan*. In this plan, you'll address, control, and change one unconscious behavior at a time, returning to Step 7 for each change you'd like to make. Ultimately, while you might not have complete control over your unconscious, your consciousness can—and, in the future, will—program the course of many of your unconscious actions.

PRE-STEP 7 QUESTIONS

Complete these questions *before* you complete the Step 7 experience.

1. **What kind of situations cause you to regress back into your unconscious ways?** What can you do to lessen the likelihood of this occurring?

2. **Where do you feel the most and least supported on your journey?** How can you gain more support moving forward? Are there ways you can acknowledge the support you've been receiving as a means of gratitude?

3. **Write a letter to your consciousness asking it to help you curate your unconscious.** Every step you've completed has led up to this one. Reflect and review on this journey and what it's been like to consciously connect and explore yourself as much as you have been.*

STEP 7 EXPERIENCE

The Step 7 experience—the creation of your *Conscious Growth Action Plan*—is a four-step process. The order of the steps are as follows: (1)

---

* For all you perfectionistic brains and humans out there, the length doesn't matter; neither does what it looks like. Just connect with yourself.

Choose the unconscious behavior you want to work on and develop its opposite conscious action, (2) assess how each part of your unconscious contributes to this behavior by answering a series of questions, (3) choose from a list (or develop your own list) of tools and techniques shown to help break habitual behaviors, and (4) begin the work of consciously curating yourself.

You will return to the Step 7 experience again and again to work on a new behavior from your *Short List*. Step 7, similar to Step 4, is one you can use to assess and adjust yourself as often as needed.

1. Conscious Growth Action Plan: To start, using your *Short List*, choose one unconscious behavior from one of your unconscious parts

CONSCIOUS GROWTH ACTION PLAN

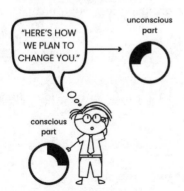

(somatic, cognitive, or psychoanalytic). Once you choose the behavior you want to change, place it in a column on one side of a piece of paper, and on the other side, write how the conscious part of you could and will handle these situations differently.

It should look something like this:

My Cognitive Unconscious	My Conscious Brain
Perfectionism: Recognizes too many details and has no coping skills to release attachment to many of them, causing delays and serious anxiety about everything	*Acceptance:* Allows minor details to exist without inspection and possesses coping skills to detach from them, leading to more timely decisions and a calmer approach

Next, evaluate the impact of each segment of your three-part unconscious on the particular unconscious trait you're aiming to improve by posing the following questions to yourself:

SOMATIC UNCONSCIOUS

1. What does it feel like *in your body* to engage in the unconscious version of this behavior?
2. What sensations do you experience that allow your unconscious to control these situations? (For example, you feel tension in your body, which makes it feel like you're doing something wrong, so you try to get it done perfectly.)
3. What would conscious "you" say your body needed in order to have more control over this behavior?

COGNITIVE UNCONSCIOUS

1. What automatic thoughts arise when engaging in this unconscious behavior?
2. Which are the thoughts you'd consider most emotional or overwhelming?
3. How do you react to these thoughts? How do you *want* to react to them?
4. What would conscious "you" say back to the unconscious thoughts attached to this behavior?

PSYCHOANALYTIC UNCONSCIOUS

1. What concepts are attached to this behavior?
2. How do your current definitions of (and the stories attached to) these concepts affect this behavior?
3. What are other ways to define these concepts that would be more helpful?

Everything we're talking about here is essentially a habit—a repetitive behavior pattern. Repeated body ignoring. Repeated thought acceptance. Repeated storytelling. In order to create good habits and break bad ones, there are very simple yet powerful tools and techniques you can apply to yourself, your environment, and your supports to maximize your chances of success. I have listed some of them here. Review the list and determine which ones you think could help grow your ability to live more consciously and more in control.

SOMATIC

Interoceptive Attunement:	Accurately perceive, interpret, and respond to your body's sensations and reactions.
Body Activation:	Engage your body as part of your process. Allow it to be positioned, tended to, and connected in the work you're doing.

COGNITIVE

Intention Setting:	Get specific, detailed, and clear when it comes to what your new behavior will look like.
First Thought, Second Thought:	Your first thought = automatic, unconscious. Your second = conscious, more reflective. Wait and listen before taking action.

PSYCHOANALYTIC

Supportive Conceptualization:	Explore the concepts and schemas related to this behavior or situation. Separate them from the meaning to see the full picture.
Storytelling:	Play the storyline through, the catastrophic one you're telling yourself in your head. Most of our stories are emotion-based and irrational. See if it's realistic.

ENVIRONMENTAL

Reduce Activation:	Minimize elements in the environment that can instigate or intensify your unconscious behavior.
Visual/Physical Cues:	Incorporate noticeable reminders or signals in the environment to reinforce and guide you.

SUPPORT

Specific Needs:	Tell your support system how they can help you with your conscious goals.
Accountability Partners:	Partner with individuals who can provide guidance and motivation to continue even when you don't want to.

In the end, each unconscious behavior you'd like to work on in Step 7 experiences should look like this—this is your *Conscious Growth Action Plan*.

Visit yourunconsciousisshowing.com/stepseven for a free downloadable Step 7 Template.

CONSCIOUS GROWTH ACTION PLAN

Unconscious Habit: Perfectionism	Conscious Goal: Acceptance
Somatic Objective: Interoceptive Attunement	I will put fifteen minutes of somatic check-in time on my calendar before each four-hour-long stretch of work to see where I'm at physically. "I will give my body what it needs at specific times."
Cognitive Objective: Metacognition	I will acknowledge that the thought "You won't be able to support your family if you slow down" is automatic and instinctual, and I don't have to listen to it. I will replace it with "You're doing, and do, great, regularly."
Psychoanalytic Objective: Storytelling	When I'm stuck on a small, unimportant aspect of my work, I will play the story out in my head (and surely come to find it's ridiculous). "If I don't get every period correctly within or outside of the parentheses, they aren't going to like the book and no one will buy it." (See *ridiculous*.)
Environmental Objective: Visual/Physical Cues	I will place a sticker on my laptop that says "Shit happens. Keep going." to remind me I am fighting the old perspective that "perfect" work is the only way to get by.
Support Objective: Accountability Partner	I will ask Max to gently point out my perfectionist tendencies when we are working on something together. I will also ask him to verbalize any moments that stand out to him about his *lack of* perfectionism and to share with me the process in his body, brain, and mind.

Your *Conscious Growth Action Plan* can be utilized in a variety of ways.

You might take on a steroid-like version of "the Serenity Prayer," dedicating thirty straight days to tackle all the goals you've set for a specific unconscious behavior. This means acknowledging when the unconscious habit occurs and vigorously addressing it with as many of your conscious goals as possible, leveraging your wisdom to know when and how to do so.

Alternatively, you could approach your goals more gradually, focusing on one every few days or adding a new objective after experiencing the positive effects of the previous one. Not every conscious effort will result in an unconscious transformation, but many will. Once you identify the actions that truly make a difference, you'll be surprised at how much easier it becomes to be in control. Trial and error. (And don't fear the error part; all potential success comes with a chance of failure.)

Step 7 is a step you should spend a significant amount of time on. The next steps involve the next phase of your interpersonal conscious work—when you'll involve others in your life again. But in order to complete these next steps, you need to have grown consciously. You need to have gained some control of your life.

Most of my clients spend around six months on this step if they are wanting to see massive change before moving on. Others—humans living a more conscious life already and/or those not dealing with heavy mental health problems—tend to spend around thirty days. They focus on one major conscious shift and then they go on.

It's up to you what you need. You know yourself (and all your parts).

Step 8: Unconscious Harms

STEP 8—Take accountability: List the people your unconscious behaviors have harmed.

Step 8 is an integral part of the 12 Steps of Consciousness.

Up to now, you've explored how your unconscious works, seen how it affects your actions, and made a plan (or maybe even several plans) to take charge of your life. Next, you're going to see how your past (and maybe even your current) unconscious actions have impacted other people.

As a clinician, and a human with an unconscious, I find it safe to say that your unconscious behaviors have without a doubt, inadvertently, if not intentionally at times, led to misunderstandings, hurts, and/or strained relationships. The truth is: Hurting people is a symptom of being alive, even if you want to pretend it's not. The difference is if that hurt is intentional, how it's handled, if it's repeated, and how much it impacts others. There's a major difference between an upsetting decision or statement and, for example, blatant, violent harm.

Step 8 gives you a proactive approach to this truth. In this step, you'll answer questions and create an *Unconscious Amends List*, one that asks you to identify and list people your unconscious has negatively affected, and the specific instances that took place.

Prepare for an emotional experience. As you list people you've hurt, an array of emotions can and likely will emerge—guilt, shame, regret. Handling these emotions consciously is crucial. We've all been unconscious, and we've all harmed people in some way. It's not necessary to make amends for simply being human. It's necessary to make amends for being a human who engaged in the act of harming people. Think action and *impact*, not just intention.

For example, say you're having an emotional day at work and, because of that, your boss moves the deadline of a project you've been working on to give you some leeway. That could technically qualify as a "yes" to question 1 from the list of questions you'll see below, which reads, "Did I make my emotions influence this person's individual decision-making?" However, this instance is not necessarily something you need to make amends for.

On the other hand, being wildly emotional and disconnected from your body and causing your (now) ex-partner to miss their college graduation ceremony because they're worried about you and your inability to care for yourself may be grounds for amends. (Note: This is not placing blame on someone who's struggling mentally or emotionally. It's acknowledging that those of us who do struggle in these ways typically *do* feel remorse for how our experiences impact the lives of others. It's okay to know you've affected others in difficult ways and admit it. You know this now.)

PRE–STEP 8 QUESTIONS

Complete these questions *before* you complete the Step 8 experience.

1. **What internal and external barriers may block your willingness to look at who you've hurt?** Sort through these now so you have the best possible chance at completing this step (and, more importantly, the next one).

2. **What values lie in listing those you have harmed?** Review your values list.

3. **In what ways have you shown yourself that you're ready to make amends?** Actions must be present to back up your words. The work you've put into seeing your unconscious ways and working to change them thus far is big. Summarize the work you completed in Steps 1 through 7. These changes are proof you know what happened in the past was wrong.

4. **What are your expectations when it comes to making amends?** What do you think are the best and worst things that could happen? What's most likely to happen?

STEP 8 EXPERIENCE

Change isn't easy. It becomes easier when you have a reason to change. Sometimes, that reason is you hurt someone, and you don't want to hurt them again. Allow yourself to grow through this experience by feeling the emotions that arise in your body as you think of the person and review the Step 8 questions. Your body's emotions are value-based. If it feels "bad," it means you recognize it as such, consciously and unconsciously. That's growth. Again, it's okay to see and show your unconscious. It's happening anyway. It's just that now, it's in your control, and you're doing something about it.

1. Unconscious Amends List: First, start by creating a list of all relevant people in your past and present, not just people you *think* you've harmed.

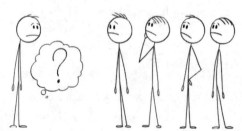

UNCONSCIOUS AMENDS LIST

This is important because you may realize your unconscious affected people you don't immediately think of as being "harmed" by you. Remember, you haven't been fully aware of yourself and your parts until now.

You can make your initial list in many ways, including listing individuals as you think of them, or you can use a system of relation, time, or location—like friends/family/

colleagues, going from elementary school to college to employment, or scanning through different cities you've lived in. If the person was in any way significant, write them down.

Once you have this first list, ask yourself questions using the list below to determine who should be included on your *Unconscious Amends List*. Read a question, then scan the names. If you arrive at a "yes" in response to a paired question and person, decide if it's important. If so, you put their name on your list so you can develop a plan for amends. If you know you should talk to them (even if you don't want to), put a check next to their name. Repeat for each question and each person.

QUESTIONS TO HELP YOU CREATE YOUR UNCONSCIOUS AMENDS LIST

1. Did I make my emotions influence this person's individual decision-making?
2. Did I make them responsible for my emotional well-being?
3. Did I disrespect their body or their sensitivities?
4. Did I make snap judgments about them?
5. Did I allow bias and selfish perspectives to determine how I treated them?
6. Did I create a concept/character I expected them to fulfill in my life?
7. Did I make my needs more important than theirs?
8. Did I force my opinions, perceptions, or decisions onto them?
9. Did I judge them for acting in ways similar to how I act?
10. Did I contribute to their helplessness or hopelessness?
11. Did I not share my needs/boundaries and blame them for how it affected me?
12. Did I assume their feelings based on what I thought and saw versus what they said and did?

Notice how the questions listed here do not involve behaviors that are objectively abusive or violent. If you've engaged in actions such as those in the past toward another person, it's likely you should be placing their name on your list.

Once you have your checked list of individuals, you can formally develop your *Unconscious Amends List*.

Use this template for each person.

UNCONSCIOUS AMENDS LIST: [NAME OF PERSON AFFECTED]

- The unconscious harm
- The opposite (conscious) action of that harm
- How the parts of my unconscious affected their life
- How the parts of my unconscious influenced our relationship
- Am I willing to make the amends? Why/why not?

Visit yourunconsciousisshowing.com/stepeight for a free downloadable Step 8 Experience Template.

POST-STEP 8 QUESTIONS

Step 8 is complete after you've made your *Unconscious Amends List*. Before starting Step 9, complete these questions as a means to reflect on and integrate your experience.

1. **What would your life be like if you already mended each of these relationships?** Envisioning a more conscious future, with more conscious relationships, helps to motivate your body and brain to keep going.

2. **Are there people on your *Unconscious Amends List* that you're angry or resentful toward?** What does your somatic unconscious have to say about those people? Can you work on managing your own internal response, the one that arises at just the thought of them, for your own sake? (Note: There may be people who have abused, neglected, or otherwise harmed you—it's *completely possible* to grow consciously without amending your relationship with them. Don't force anything that doesn't make sense.)

I know Step 8 can hurt. It doesn't feel good to acknowledge the harm we've done, especially when much of our pain often goes unacknowledged by others. And you did it. Congratulations. Your journey to consciousness isn't isolated; it's intertwined with the experiences, emotions, and lives of those around you. By developing a list of harms you're responsible for, by striving to mend and heal, you won't just elevate yourself, you'll uplift and support those around you. It's okay to want to be better than you once were, and there's nothing wrong with telling that to people you once hurt.

Step 9: Acts of Amends

STEP 9—Actively amend your unconscious interpersonal harms.

When you're growing consciously, the weight of your unconscious and harmful actions can be overwhelming. Step 9 offers you a chance to lighten this load. You do not exist alone, therefore you do not heal alone.

There are three different types of amends you will offer others throughout this step—Direct Amends, Indirect Amends, and Living Amends.

Direct Amends: This is the crux of the Step 9 experience. Here, you will directly address and resolve past harms through face-to-face conversations and tangible action—like offering to help lighten the load of someone who needed your support in the past but you were too busy conceptualizing them, expecting and demanding them to "figure it out themselves." (I see this a lot with parents, partners, bosses, and siblings.)

Indirect Amends: If direct amends are not possible or may cause harm—for example, if bringing up old harms would interfere with someone's new relationship or life functioning or if they aren't reachable—then you instead make amends through corrective action. This includes things like contributing positively to a community or group of people you once harmed or engaging in acts of service toward those similar to this person (like working at a food bank in a community of people who you once considered to be less than you). You do not need to inform them of why you're helping them (unless it would better their lives to know the story of your past harms toward the person you cannot directly show amends to and support).

Living Amends: By controlling your life using the 12 Steps of Consciousness, you're dedicating your time, energy, and efforts toward not harming others in the future in the same way you did the person on your amends list. This third option is something that should be a constant, with direct or indirect amends being the priority.

Now, to put it lightly, this path isn't always smooth. People's reactions can vary, from understanding to outright rejection. (I've been rejected during this step. It's difficult, and we get through it.)

The key to successful completion of Step 9 is to be genuine, ready to listen, and prepared for any response. As you probably know, when humans are hurt, we consciously and unconsciously change. We hold resentments, blame, hurt, pain, and can express these emotions, thoughts, and feelings when they arise (even if we don't mean to).

Be sure you're mentally ready to take care of yourself no matter the outcome. Your unconscious will try and protect you—it will give you reasons to fear the conversation, reasons to change your mind, and reasons to not do something without knowing the outcome will be a "good" one.

Consciously control your unconscious. Make your own decisions. **You are in control.**

STEP 9 EXPERIENCE

When working your way down your *Unconscious Amends List*, feel free to start with either your most difficult amends or the one you believe to be the easiest. Keep in mind that this is not about you experiencing a shift in how someone feels about you or what you did—it's not about forgiveness. It's about you acknowledging and acting in accordance with your conscious values, whether they forgive you or not.

1. Acts of Amends: For this exercise, take your *Unconscious Amends List* from Step 8 and hold a meaningful, selfless conversation with the person you harmed.

An important piece of this experience is that you hold conversations with one person at a time, even if it's a group of individuals you'd like to address.

DIRECT AMENDS

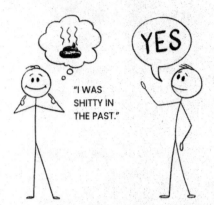

Each person involved has their own body, brain, and mind that was affected by your unconscious. You both deserve time and space to discuss the experience with open and active ears and hearts.

Visit yourunconsciousisshowing.com/stepnine for a free downloadable Step 9 Experience Template.

Use this breakdown for your Direct Amends process:

- **Nature of Amends:** Identify what form your amends should take. Is it a verbal apology, written letter, gesture, or perhaps a combination?
- **Setting:** Determine a suitable setting for making amends. It should be comfortable and conducive to open communication. If in-person isn't viable, would a phone call or video chat be appropriate? Ensure the person you're seeking to provide amends to will be comfortable.
- **Practice:** Before approaching the person, practice what you plan to say with someone you trust or even in front of a mirror. This helps in refining your message and ensuring it's sincere and clear.
- **Self-reflection:** Recognize and acknowledge your feelings about this step. Are there fears, reservations, or anxieties? Write them down. Assess your unconscious.
- **Affirmations:** Create a set of positive affirmations to reassure yourself. Example: "I am undertaking this step to heal, grow, and make right what was wrong."
- **Active Listening:** Be prepared to listen more than you speak. Understand their feelings and perspectives without getting defensive. (This one is *so* key. Know your boundaries, and control your responses. You're more conscious now, remember?)

> - **Acceptance:** Understand that the outcome isn't always in your control. Be prepared for a range of reactions. Accept what you cannot control, and control what you can. This is the work.
> - **Gratitude:** Regardless of the outcome, acknowledge and appreciate your courage in taking this step, and their willingness to attempt to hear you out. Remember, it's about growth and healing. We are all trying our best. We are all human first.

POST–STEP 9 QUESTIONS

Complete these questions *after* you complete the Step 9 experience.

1. **How did your first amends feel?** What was the response? What lessons emerged?

2. **After several attempts at making amends, what are your key takeaways?** Were there recurring themes? Were there unexpected or disappointing outcomes?

3. **How has the process of making amends influenced how you handle new relationships you enter into?** Making amends can suck. The goal is to act in ways where amends are no longer needed.

4. **How are you processing feedback post-amends?** How is your unconscious? How are you resisting the urge to justify your actions and stay the conscious course?

5. **What steps are you taking to make amends to yourself?** You didn't forget to include yourself on your list, did you?! You matter too, you know. Spend time here. Do you forgive yourself? Could you forgive yourself? *Will you?*
   - **Bonus:** Write your consciousness a letter of amends for not acknowledging it for so long.
   - **Extra Bonus:** Write an apology to your unconscious for making it exist alone, without conscious direction.

6. **What specific amends have sharpened your understanding of the damage you caused?** How have these insights boosted your humility?

The wrongs you've amended, and will continue to amend, may be some of the heaviest anchors that have kept you trapped, distant from a conscious existence. One of the greatest gifts I find that comes from Step 9 is experiencing more of an interest in the feelings and thoughts of other people, being less selfish. It hurts to admit where we went wrong, and that's not an excuse to keep someone else hurting.

As I say, we are *constantly* in relationships instead of being *consciously* in them. Making amends is how we experience and cultivate stronger, more conscious relationships. Be proud of yourself. This step is not about forgiveness. It's about understanding what happened, how it made them feel, and moving in ways that make the world a less painful place.

Steps 5 through 9 wrap up the core journey in the 12 Steps of Consciousness. You've shared your unconscious with another human being, put into action a plan for conscious living, and addressed the unintended impacts of your past behaviors. Now, as you move into the final chapter of the book and the next phase of your life, the journey changes.

Steps 10 to 12 are maintenance steps. They'll keep you on the path of consciousness and guide you in creating a more conscious world. Don't forget the skills and strategies you've picked up in the first nine steps. Use them regularly to stay in tune with the most conscious version of "you" that you can.

You may still have ninety-nine problems, but now your unconscious isn't one.

CHAPTER 8 SUMMARY

- You have a past. That doesn't mean you can't do a full twist and start changing and controlling your life.
- Showing your unconscious to another human is as vulnerable as it is necessary—Step 5.
- The middle of your consciousness journey is where the work begins. It gets real when you create a list of self-chosen "cons"—Step 6.
- Batman is a human and you have a superpower just like him. The work continues when you force your unconscious to change—Step 7.
- All humans hurt other humans, even if only unconsciously, unintentionally. It's okay to admit that—Step 8.
- You can't grow consciously without mending the pain your unconscious has given others—Step 9.

9

Go In and Give Back

Growth and Service, Steps 10, 11, and 12

Throughout history, defining the line between life and death has challenged society, medicine, and the hearts of many human beings. In 1990, Terri, a young woman from Florida, experienced a heart attack and brain injury, entered into a vegetative state, and was placed in an extreme life-or-death situation—one that would rattle the country for over fifteen years.[1]

A "vegetative state" is a state of living where you experience *wakefulness without awareness*[2]—where you appear to be awake and your eyes may even be open, but you lack any form of conscious response. Terri was "awake" but showed no perceivable signs of "consciousness." It was assumed her unconscious was controlling 100 percent of her body and brain—breathing, circulation, and any and all responses and movements. She remained in this state for eight years, at which time her husband, Michael, petitioned to have her feeding tube removed. His petition led to a protracted legal and emotional battle between himself and her parents, Bob and Mary.

Michael fought for a "compassionate end" to Terri's life—one that stopped her artificial life support (and, in Michael's eyes, her potential suffering). On the other hand, Terri's parents believed she could recover and that the medical interventions keeping her "alive" should be maintained. The dispute between the two parties lasted seven years, involved numerous court battles, and included intense discussions around things like medical malpractice, estate inheritance, and the Roman Catholic Church's teachings. The case was so emotional and divisive that it eventually required intervention from both the United States Congress and President George W. Bush.

The final court decision was to side with Michael and allow Terri's feeding tube to be removed. She was pronounced dead on March 31, 2005. After over fifteen years without objective consciousness and almost two weeks without her feeding tube, Terri's unconscious could no longer sustain her life on its own.

Terri experienced twenty-six years of consciousness. During that time, she met Michael while attending community college; they fell in love and chose to live in Florida in order to live near her parents, whom she also loved. She worked as an insurance bookkeeper. Terri's gravestone reads, "Departed This Earth February 25, 1990"—the day she lost her ability to be conscious—not the date in 2005 when her heart irreversibly stopped and her brain died.[3]

To Michael, his wife's life ended the day she stopped being conscious. The day her unconscious had 100 percent control over her. The day there was nothing she could do to consciously change or control her life.

Determining the legal, philosophical, and ethical dimensions of death when it comes to medical decisions is still up for debate—and not one I'm particularly interested in getting myself too involved in. However, there is one accepted definition of **death** I want you to know, and it's this:

Death is the permanent stopping of all critical life functions—respiration, circulation, homeostasis-related functions . . . and *consciousness*.[4]

Terri's clinical diagnosis, "wakefulness without awareness," or a vegetative state, can have reversible or permanent forms.[5] It can be hard to tell which form someone is experiencing, hence the battle between her husband and parents. Humans have a hard time accepting brain death as the end, and we should, because we don't *really* know if the person's inner thoughts and feelings are gone, too. Our consciousness is only our own. No one else can truly know it, remember?

At the time of my writing this book, there are no tests proving that brain activity seen in people in a vegetative state *isn't* them *being conscious of* and *experiencing* what's happening. It might be, and they just can't tell us. It might not be, and they may truly be gone. The only person who knew if Terri was actually conscious or not was Terri.

The point of the story is this: The only person who can truly say if *you* are conscious or not, who can decide if you have consciousness and are engaging consciously with the world, is *you*.

So, I ask you this, having made it through the first nine Steps of Consciousness:

Are you *alive*?

Pause and think about it.

Are you *conscious*?

If you're *thinking*, must you be? (Welcome to philosophy.)

Are you *engaging in the essence of human life*?

While those may be difficult questions to answer, be grateful you get to be the one to answer them. Be grateful you can communicate what is and is not in your control. Be grateful these questions are being asked to you in a *meaningful* way, not a medical way.

When it comes to determining how much your unconscious is showing and how much you're able to make conscious decisions, there are no court debates involving subjects of religion, greed, or ethics. You don't have to get the American government involved (thankfully). The power struggle between your unconscious and consciousness is not permanent. It's reversible. And the journey you're on doesn't have to take the next fifteen years of your life.

The task you're given now that you've reached the last chapter of this book and the final three steps is not to determine if you're conscious or unconscious like Terri's family was for her—you're both. You've done the work. You know this well now.

Your task is to make the relationship between all your parts finally *mean something*, because your life hasn't ended like Terri's or almost ended like Anita and her near-death experience. Right now, your unconscious doesn't have 100 percent control over you. You *are* conscious, you *are* changing, and **you are in control**. Tell yourself that. And tell everyone else, too.

Step 10: Ongoing Self-Consciousness

STEP 10—Enlighten yourself regularly; unconscious patterns are powerful.

Personal growth is not automatic; it demands effort, attention, and planning.

Step 10 is the beginning of learning how to *maintain* your consciousness. During regular intervals in your life (let's say every six months), you will review your values, emotions, thoughts, feelings, perceptions, and behaviors, to see what you've done, how you feel about it, and if you need to change or take back control. As a human, you're bound to make mistakes. Anticipate them.

In Step 10, you will complete a *Conscious Human Self-Assessment*, once now and then ongoing, twice a year. The goal of these assessments is to help you not regress back into your old, unconscious ways, keeping your path to consciousness clear, and if not clear, at least reflected upon.

Just as a gardener doesn't merely plant seeds, water them a few times, and walk away, expecting them to grow without care, you can't assume that your journey toward consciousness is complete after just addressing your past, enacting change, and making amends. The garden of your body, brain, and mind require regular tending. Continuously monitor your thoughts, feelings, and behaviors. Be vigilant.

When you see your unconscious showing, even in mild to moderate ways, promptly acknowledge it, listen to it. By doing this, you prevent small missteps from growing into larger, more complex problems, and reinforce your commitment to a conscious life. This might mean making amends, altering a decision, or simply acknowledging the lapse and setting an intention to avoid it in the future. Sorrys along with actions can go a long way.

Conscious Human Self-Assessments aren't just about figuring out where you went wrong in the prior six months. They're also about seeing the wins and looking forward to experiencing more in the future. The steps have put you through a lot of highs and lows so far. Review your progress, too.

Keep getting better. You can do this.

PRE-STEP 10 QUESTIONS

Complete these questions *before* you begin the Step 10 experience.

1. **Why is it important to you to check in with your consciousness level?** Give it purpose. Give it meaning.
2. **How do you want to complete your semiannual assessments?** Solo or with a companion or accountability partner? In writing or in discussion? Electronic or in a journal? Why?
3. **What would make you unconsciously forget (or intentionally refuse) to complete these assessments?** Why? Knowing what will get in the way helps reduce the probability that it will.
4. **What is your plan to ensure you complete your Conscious Human Self-Assessments?** Perhaps calendar alerts, scheduling them on easy-to-remember dates, etc.
5. **What is going to distract you from consciousness over the next six months?** What are you going to do about it?

STEP 10 EXPERIENCE

Complete these questions as thoughtfully and truthfully as possible. The more raw and real, the better you'll feel!

Visit yourunconsciousisshowing.com/stepten for a free downloadable Step 10 Experience Template.

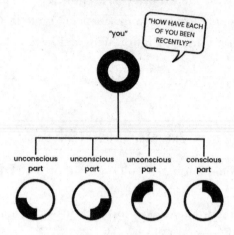

CONSCIOUS HUMAN SELF-ASSESSMENT

1. If your somatic unconscious could talk, what would it say about how you've listened to, cared for, and treated it over the last six months? Note the good and bad.

2. If you had to choose a Vibe Check level for the last six months, what would you choose?

3. What are the big decisions you made over the last six months? Were they conscious or unconscious?

4. What unconscious judgments and biases did you engage in?

5. What was your best conscious moment? Your best unconscious one?

6. What was your worst unconscious moment? Your worst conscious one?

7. In what ways did your unconscious serve you?

8. How did being a conscious human make you better over this time period?

9. Who do you need to make amends to and why? Will you? Why or why not?

10. What do you need to accept about your unconscious during this time period?

11. What are the values and concepts driving your life right now?

12. What are you doing to continue to grow consciously daily?

13. What do you have to be grateful for right now? List at least three things. And then allow the gratitude to settle into your body, and pick one thing you can do to acknowledge and/or help what you're grateful for. (Most people stop at the list and miss the action part of gratitude.)

Step 11: Furthering Your Conscious Understanding

STEP 11—Continuously expand and adjust your understanding of consciousness.

The six blind men at the beginning of this book debated the concept of an elephant.

Humans have been debating what consciousness and the unconscious are, their purpose, function, and controllability for . . . ever, really. As much as we have defined *truths* as human beings, we still falter, and will continue to, because there are big questions about this existence we can't answer—like *why* are we conscious? What is the point of life? Is there any *true* reality we could all come to realize one day? These are questions that drive us absolutely insane. (Questions I plan to answer in my next book.)

Religion, spirituality, cultural traditions, and other forms of creative and meaningful human development have attempted to answer these fundamental questions for us, as have scientists, researchers, and clinicians of the human condition. Their work is important. It's what allowed me to share the wisdom found within this book.

However, you cannot and should not expect that what you gain from this book is enough to understand your place on this planet, your level of consciousness, or the true depths of your unconscious.

More learning is always required. Why? Because you weren't born conscious. At least not in the meaningful sense.

On day one, if you were lucky, you were born alive and breathing on your own. But, at the moment of birth, you're not truly *awake*. Not truly *present* to yourself, your inner and outer circumstances, and to what it *means* to experience life. When you're little, you're experiencing aliveness, awareness, and presence, but it has no inherent meaning, at least not one you're conscious of.

Then suddenly, at times step-by-step, things start to change.

A moment happens. A day happens. A year happens. Something beautiful. Sometimes devastating. Unexpected, or perhaps deeply desired. Moments like your child being born, finding out your partner is cheating on you, or realizing you're unconscious and can do something about it. Now, you're conscious in a *meaningful* way. You feel more alive, more aware, than ever—whether you like it or not.

The first time being a *conscious* human being actually *meant* something to me, I was sitting in a small shed in the back of the Malibu rehab center I worked at, crying my eyes out. Two years into my ultimatum-triggered healing journey in 2012, and I was about to realize the unconscious was the biggest part of the human experience I was missing.

The day prior, I had said something to my supervisor about how I felt like I "didn't have any empathy"[6]—even though I was training to become a therapist. Jaymee Carpenter, the spiritual director of the facility, overheard our conversation and asked if I would be willing to partake in a short meditative exercise during my lunch break the next day. Jaymee didn't believe I lacked empathy. He believed I lacked conscious awareness of my own feelings (and knowledge of what feelings even were).

I reluctantly (and I mean *reluctantly*) agreed.

"Come with me to meet Courtney," Jaymee said, as he motioned his hand toward himself while walking out the door. He was always attempting to sound and seem profoundly deep, and to be fair, he nailed it almost every single time. I followed him down a small dirt hill in the back of the house, one lined with crooked wooden stairs, to the shed where I would, in fact, "meet myself" for the first time (honestly, I was still rolling my eyes at this point).

We sat in two chairs, about seven feet apart, facing each other. It was serious. The entire shed was only around fifteen feet long and ten feet wide. It was meant to be storage for the facility's gardening equipment and had a dreamy view of the Pacific Ocean and some of the world's most sought-after vacation beaches. It was the kind of location you find yourself in and ask: How did I end up in such a beautiful location, hiding inside a shed at work finding out who the fuck I am at twenty-four years old? (When therapists say we've been where our clients are, we mean it.)

The exercise Jaymee walked me through was called a Metta Meditation. This form of meditation is a traditional Buddhist practice meant to cultivate *metta*, a "mental state of positive energy and kindness toward oneself and other beings, as opposed to the anger, hostility, or self-loathing that often accompany emotional problems."[7] This practice has also been shown to be effective for borderline personality disorder,[8] the symptomatology I was working on reducing at the time (although Jaymee did not know that).

"Let's start by having you focus on your body."

Oh, shit. I was panicking already. I always felt uncomfortable, anxious, and in pain. I did not want to feel a damn thing. But the guided, slow, deep breathing he walked me through helped.

"You're probably hearing lots of thoughts in your head. Let them pass," he said.

Does he know I'm panicking and my thoughts are going a million miles an hour? Are his eyes open, watching me? Do I look weird doing this? How much longer is this going to be? His telling me that I am not my thoughts allowed me to detach from them for the time being.

"Now, while holding on to the awareness of your body and your thoughts, bring little Courtney to the forefront of your mind." An image of five-year-old me popped into my head. Tears immediately started trailing down my face. (I really hoped he wasn't looking at me.)

Dead. He had killed the current version of who I was in that moment, in just a single moment. I would never be the same. Sounds dramatic, and if you know, you know. When you first realize how much of yourself you've been missing, it's almost like your life starts all over again. It's such a heavy grief.

I don't remember how long I was able to stay connected to little Courtney, but it was the first time I allowed myself to see "me" like that, and it changed my life. It wasn't about healing an actual "inner child"; rather, it was about correcting how I'd been connecting with my unconscious—"Little Courtney" was just a metaphor, a conceptual IKEA room, containing the messages from my body, my brain's automatic patterns and thoughts, and the way they both shaped my life experiences through the stories I'd been telling myself for over twenty years. I was, and am, all of the stories, all of the parts, including the concept of little Courtney.

My first conscious moment wasn't something devastating or shocking—at least nothing compared to the January 2019 incident that catapulted me into The Truth Doctor. But it was unexpected. Being conscious—having the ability to go inward and learn about my unconscious—finally *meant something*. It became a real tool and superpower I had, but never knew I had. Until then.

Jaymee changed my life that day—so much so that I asked him to officiate my wedding with Max because, without this experience, I never would have been able to love my husband as deeply as I am able to now.*

My *Metta* experience was the beginning of what I like to call **meaningful consciousness.**

Meaningful consciousness is more than just being alive. It's more than just being aware. It's more than the type of possible consciousness that shows up in the brain scans of people in a vegetative state like Terri.

Meaningful consciousness is controlled consciousness; it's intentional consciousness.

It's using consciousness to explore into your unconscious, build connections with others, and guide society and your generation toward a positive, human existence.

My past: I always had feelings. I ignored their meaning. I always had thoughts. I gave them too much meaning. I always had experiences. I focused more on what I didn't like about them than what I did, more on what was out of my control than what was in it.

I was a passive, helpless, chained passenger on a journey toward wherever my unconscious wanted to take me. The shocks became

---

* P.S. For those who have made it to the final chapter in this book: I also officiate weddings, so email me if I end up changing your life, and I'll officiate yours. Jaymee does too, and he offers counseling. Look him up.

normalized. I had never given myself the chance to control my consciousness, to allow consciousness to bring me joy, insight, connection, love, balance, and self-awareness. Self-consciousness was a bad
thing in my world and went no deeper than my skin.

That day, with Jaymee, changed everything for me.

Throughout these two final Steps of Consciousness, Steps 11 and
12, you get the opportunity to do for someone else what Jaymee did
for me, and what I hope I have done for you by writing this book and
telling my truth to help you find yours.

Step 11 is where you're asked to widen your perspective on what it
means to be "conscious," and to understand the unconsciousness that
lives within you, me, and all of us.

To grow as a conscious individual, you need to grasp your place
within a larger context, the larger world, and our planet's population
of eight billion people. This means acknowledging the balance between
your personal introspections and the education available to you from
other sources—similarly to how the blind men came to realize they
needed to combine their truths to understand the true essence of the
elephant and how you combined each part of your unconscious to truly
see it showing.

On one hand, self-reflection helps you understand your thoughts and
actions. On the other, seeking external wisdom—from books, mentors,
or professionals—can and will enhance your personal understanding. I
was two years into my healing journey when this afternoon with Jaymee
took place. I was self-reflecting already. But I needed a new understanding. One I could only get from someone else.

Step 11's experiences guide you through a kaleidoscope of personal, social, cultural, and spiritual experiences to help you see consciousness from various angles and perspectives. Part of this step, for
me, as a human and a healer, has always been about seeking to better
understand existence and consciousness on a foundational level. I
constantly find myself asking: **"Why do I exist and how can I, a conscious human being, make it mean something?"**

The more you learn about yourself, the unconscious, and consciousness, the more this question seems to become answerable. It's worth

making finding the answer to this question your purpose in life. I made it mine, and it's been exceedingly worthwhile.

STEP 11 QUESTIONS

1. **How has your understanding of "consciousness" and "the unconscious" changed since being on this journey?** Not comparing before to right now, but how it's changed *incrementally* throughout the steps.

2. **How did you expect to continue learning about consciousness before reaching Step 11?** Your answer can help you gauge what your unconscious thought was going to work (or that it wasn't thinking about it at all).

3. **What are your favorite sources of wisdom and knowledge about mental health, wellness, humanity, and consciousness?** If you don't have any, start by joining my social communities (@the.truth.doctor). I constantly share sources there.

4. **How has your concept of "you" been altered by your conscious growth? In what ways has it stayed the same?**

STEP 11 EXPERIENCE

You have five choices. You can venture into all, or just gravitate toward the one that resonates the most. The first one is the meditation Jaymee walked me though. Remember, every time you engage in one of these experiences, you're making a conscious choice toward more self-awareness and heightened consciousness.

Visit yourunconsciousisshowing.com/stepeleven for a free downloadable Step 11 Experience Template.

1. Metta Meditation: Place yourself in a comfortable seated or lying

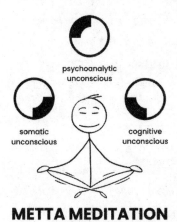

psychoanalytic
unconscious

somatic
unconscious

cognitive
unconscious

METTA MEDITATION

down position with your back straight or flat, feet on the ground or out straight, and arms gently in your lap or folded over your heart. Breathe naturally, focusing on your breathing for a short while (a couple of minutes or so). If focusing on your breath is too much, practice focusing on your body as a whole or on a specific place in your view and gently giving it your attention.

When you're ready, read each of the prompts below, one at a time.

Picture yourself sitting alone during a past age. You decide the age, whichever one comes up for you initially. Watch yourself. Try to connect to the emotions, thoughts, perceptions, and conceptualizations living within and around this version of you. When you're ready (after a few minutes of conscious observation and sensation), say these words in your mind or out loud to past you: *May you be happy, may you be healthy, may you be safe, and may you be at ease.*

Now bring to mind someone you love. Picture them smiling at you. Imagine what they say to you and how they make you feel. What feelings arise in them when they see you? Experience the connection you've built with them. When you're ready, say these words to them: *May you be happy, may you be healthy, may you be safe, and may you be at ease.*

Next, bring to mind a neutral person in your life. Someone you see regularly, but don't have a relationship with—like a local barista you see often or a school crosswalk guard or the receptionist at your workplace. Imagine what their life may be like, how they have the same amount of experiences you do daily, along with hopes, dreams, fears, and probably a similar desire for more sleep and less stress.

Picture them smiling at you and repeat these words again: *May you be happy, may you be healthy, may you be safe, and may you be at ease.*

Now, picture a person who has done you harm in the past. It does not have to be a person who caused you extreme pain. It can be someone who upset you or caused a moderate delay or mild rupture in your life, to start. (Eventually, it's helpful to expand this practice to those who have deeply hurt you, but that takes significant time.) Picture them with a neutral facial expression, one that allows you to see them as human. When you're ready, repeat these words: *May they be happy, may they be healthy, may they be safe, and may they be at ease.*

*Notice how I did not ask you to see them smiling at you. Don't force something unnatural.

Lastly, widen your vision to all human beings on planet Earth. Imagine, if just for a moment, what it would be like for us all to coexist, consciously and intentionally, on our planet. Spend time here, it's good for the soul. And when you're ready, I invite you to repeat these words again: *May we be happy, may we be healthy, may we be safe, and may we be at ease.*

Write down your reflections.

2. Yoga or Another Body-Based Movement: Incorporate yoga or another form of physical activity, like tai chi, dance, light stretching, or a short daily walk (about twenty minutes) into your daily routine. Pay attention to how your breathing syncs up with your movements, and notice how your body's sensations connect with your thoughts. Choose a challenging pose or speed and hold it a little longer each day. This practice will enhance your awareness and grow your control.

BODY-BASED MOVEMENT

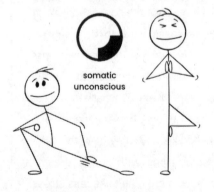

somatic unconscious

Purposeful physical activities use concentration, awareness, and clear thinking. As you get better at certain poses, sequences, or speeds, you're training the parts of your unconscious that handle routines, memories, and learned behaviors to listen to "you" more.

3. Conscious Learning and Exploration: Make a continuous effort to learn about consciousness and all three parts of the unconscious. This might mean reading books, watching videos, or going to talks and workshops that cover various areas of these concepts—like neuroscience content about automatic cognition or a fact-checked blog about how grief changes your eating and sleeping patterns. By introducing yourself to new ideas, theories, and viewpoints, you reshape and expand your cognitive conceptualizations.

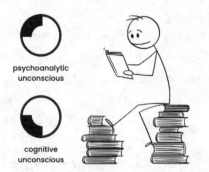

LEARNING AND EXPLORATION

psychoanalytic unconscious

cognitive unconscious

Bonus: Create a journal of insights, questions, or reflections that arise. Consider sharing or discussing these in study groups, online forums, or social media.

4. Community and/or Spiritual Engagement: Start or join a group focused on sharing and discussing personal journeys of consciousness, possibly even working through the 12 Steps of Consciousness as a group. Exchange stories and thoughts; they will give you deeper understanding of your own and others' deep-seated unconscious processes. Get involved in discussions, debates, or group learning that challenges your existing ways of thinking.

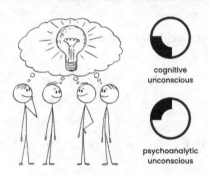

COMMUNITY ENGAGEMENT

cognitive unconscious

psychoanalytic unconscious

Bonus: Initiate or participate in community events that align with growing consciousness, such as community meditations, awareness campaigns, or consciousness-based workshops.

5. Conscious Cultural Expansion: Dedicate time to immersing yourself in a culture different from your own. Eat their food, listen to their music, read about their traditions. Experiencing different cultures grows your understanding of the diverse world around you. You'll be amazed at how other cultures view consciousness, existence, control, and responsibility. When you're ready, take it further by engaging in a conversation with someone from another culture, with the intention of expanding your conceptual understanding of life, existence, and *being human*. We are all the same, yet we are all so different.

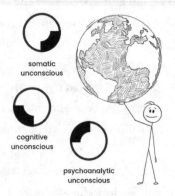

CONSCIOUS CULTURAL EXPANSION

somatic unconscious

cognitive unconscious

psychoanalytic unconscious

Bonus: Engage in cultural exchange programs, learn a new language, or partake in international seminars and workshops focusing on global perspectives.

Step 12: Shared Consciousness

STEP 12—Grown consciously? Good.
Now, help someone else do the same.

Being "The Truth Doctor"—someone people message daily with appreciation and gratitude for helping them improve their lives—is not who I ever expected to be. As someone who lived unconsciously for the majority of her life, leading by action was the least of my life goals. I wished to never be seen, let alone to see myself.

What I've come to learn over the last five years since I started this Truth Doctor journey is that the paradoxes I shared with you in Chapter Six are as true as they possibly could be: The more you accept you're unconscious, the less unconscious you become, and the more you admit being a human is hard, the easier it becomes to be one.

Seemingly, my most valuable contributions to others arise when I'm fully "Courtney," and not some conceptualized version of what anyone thinks I should be, whether that's as a "therapist," "mom," or "wife." I'm the most helpful when I'm human, first. I'm the most helpful when I share my story and the lessons I've learned along the way. This is how you can be helpful, too.

There are many ways to share your journey, your story, your consciousness (and your unconscious) with others. The first is through a way similar to how I do it on the internet—share with others who you are as a human, before all else, and don't be afraid to admit your unconscious is showing, making repairs quickly. This is *Leading By Action*.

You don't have to do this on the internet. You can do it with your friends, your colleagues, your kids, your partner. Sharing that which has helped you heal, to help others heal, is what every single person has done who has changed the world or someone's life for the better.

The second is to be a *Conscious Support*—someone who guides another person through the 12 Steps of Consciousness. There might be people who've noticed your transformation and are not only intrigued by your growth but who have also shown a desire to embark on the 12 Steps themselves. This is how we grow a more conscious world.

You are ready to extend a helping hand to those starting their conscious path. The first eleven steps led you here. Through your actions (informed by your insights, acceptance, courage, and wisdom) you will become a *beacon of light* for those observing and learning from you. As Paulo Coelho says, "No one lights a lamp in order to hide it behind the door: the purpose of light is to create more light, to open people's eyes, to reveal the marvels around." You can help someone see themselves, without a filter. You can help them be self-conscious, in a good way.

PRE-STEP 12 QUESTIONS

Complete these questions *before* you begin the Step 12 experience.

1. How has your new level of consciousness rubbed off on others around you?
2. How has your life come to be more "conscious" overall?
3. What do you wish you did differently during your 12 Steps of Consciousness?
4. What are you grateful took place along your 12-Step path?
5. What do you say to people who mention "consciousness" or "the unconscious" now that you've experienced the 12 Steps?
6. Overall, how did the 12 Steps of Consciousness change your life?

STEP 12 EXPERIENCE

This process requires mindfulness, patience, and respect for others', as well as your own, boundaries. Recognize and respect the individuality of each person's journey by listening to them and gently guiding them, not controlling their conscious experience or their 12-Step journey. While your insights are valuable, everyone must discover their own path and walk their own walk.

Visit yourunconsciousisshowing.com/steptwelve for a free downloadable Step 12 Experience Template.

1. Conscious Support: For this exercise, you will be a supportive person in

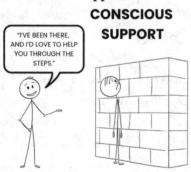

CONSCIOUS SUPPORT

"I'VE BEEN THERE, AND I'D LOVE TO HELP YOU THROUGH THE STEPS."

the life of someone walking themselves through the 12 Steps of Consciousness, as you did. Your relationship with them in terms of intensity depends on what's needed. However, as this is a significantly introspective journey, much of their path must be walked alone, as was yours. You cannot have their experiences for them nor answer their questions. You cannot know their consciousness. Simply support them as a human being who understands the struggle of controlling your three-part unconscious. You got through it and they can, too.

Use this as a guide to your *Conscious Support* process:

- **Self-Reflection:** Before seeking to guide another, spend some time reflecting on your own journey through the 12 Steps. Recall the challenges you faced, the revelations you had, and the tools or strategies that were most beneficial. This will serve as foundational knowledge in your mentorship role.

- **Initial Meeting:** Your initial meeting should be a safe space for open dialogue. Start by sharing a brief overview of your journey without diving too deep into specifics—just enough to build trust and rapport. Allow them to share their motivations and apprehensions.

- **Establish Boundaries:** Discuss and set clear boundaries regarding communication frequency, meeting times, and the nature of the relationship. Ensure both parties are comfortable and in agreement.

- **Step-by-Step Guidance:** As they progress through each step, offer your insights and experiences relevant to that particular step. Always ensure your guidance is suggestive rather than prescriptive, allowing them to find their own understanding and path.

- **Continuous Feedback:** After every few steps, set aside time for feedback. Let them express what they found beneficial, what challenges they faced, and how you might better support them.

- **Celebrate Milestones:** Each completed step is an achievement. Celebrate these milestones with them, whether it's simply acknowledging their progress or having a small celebration.

- **Handle Challenges with Empathy:** They will face challenges, just as you did. When these arise, approach them with understanding. Share how you overcame similar challenges, but also encourage them to find their solutions.

> • **Closure:** Once they complete all 12 Steps, have a final meeting. Reflect on the journey, discuss their transformation, and talk about the future. Encourage them to become a conscious support themselves, ensuring the cycle of knowledge sharing and conscious growth continues.

Conclusion

As we come to a close, I hope you feel as though you've consciously changed. I hope you feel like you have more control over yourself and your life than you once felt you did. And I hope you understand yourself better as a human being. One with a body, brain, and mind that deserves to be understood, respected, and cared for.

Being an unconscious human is something you never have to do alone again. I'm here, and so is every other reader of this book. So is every other person working the 12 Steps of Consciousness. They're out there. Go find them.

Growing consciously is a necessary, step-by-step process—one that, if we continue to share, I'm sure can save the world. Until next time, I'm Dr. Courtney, and remember: Your unconscious is showing, but it's okay, *so is everybody else's.*

CHAPTER 9 SUMMARY

- You can decide how conscious you are. It's more of a privilege than you may think.
- Get self-conscious. Over and over again. At least twice a year—Step 10.
- You know your consciousness. Get to know others' consciousness, too. There's so much you don't know and deserve to learn—Step 11.
- Lead by action and consciously support others. It's actually pretty simple—Step 12.
- You're right. Being a human is hard. And you're doing fucking fantastic.

"It seems like the chaos of this world is accelerating, but so is the beauty in the consciousness of more and more people." —Anthony Kiedis

The 12 Steps of Consciousness and Therapeutic Evidence-Based Alignment

In this book, I have suggested several different "experiences" within the 12 Steps of Consciousness. These experiences are meant to serve as a basis for your consciousness work. While the 12 Steps of Consciousness themselves are not evidence-based, almost every experience included in the 12-Step process is rooted in clinically sound modalities and practices. However, this does not mean every experience will be beneficial or adaptive for your specific situation.

Your level of consciousness and the strength and development of your three-part unconscious, as you've learned, are highly affected by what you experience in life—abuse, neglect, other traumas, genetics, neurodevelopmental conditions, chronic and acute physical illness and disorders, mental illness, socioeconomic and cultural factors, and more will all affect how the experiences feel for you. You are your own individual human.

Most experiences can be aligned with more than one modality, although I have only chosen one modality per experience. The purpose of this section is to allow you to see the potential outcomes desired for each individual step experience.

Note: Aligning the 12 Steps of Consciousness experiences with therapeutic modalities does not mean you are engaging in therapy while completing them. Therapy is a specific type of support that involves a therapist–client relationship, and to engage in these evidence-based modalities would involve informed consent and, in many cases, the following of specific manualized treatment protocols.

Step	Experience	Therapeutic Evidence-Based Alignment
Step 1: Admit it	1. Unconscious List 2. Consequences List 1/2. Motivational Interviewing (MI)	Why: MI is about eliciting change by helping clients recognize the negative consequences of their current behaviors and the potential benefits of change. By outlining the consequences of unconscious choices, individuals can be more motivated to change these behaviors, aligning with the principles of MI.
Step 2 Believe in yourself	1. Body Scan Meditation 2. Delayed Emotional Gratification Test 3. Concept Development Recall	1. Mindfulness-Based Stress Reduction (MBSR) and Mindfulness-Based Cognitive Therapy (MBCT) Why: Both of these therapies incorporate the body scan as a core mindfulness practice. The body scan meditation helps individuals become more aware of physical sensations, promoting grounding and present-moment awareness. It can be particularly useful in recognizing stress and tension. 2. Dialectical Behavior Therapy (DBT) Why: One of the core skills taught in DBT is distress tolerance, which trains individuals to accept and tolerate distress without acting impulsively. The exercise of delaying emotional responses aligns with this skill, teaching individuals to sit with their emotions without reacting immediately.

		3. Psychoanalytic/Psychodynamic Therapy Why: This approach delves into past experiences and unconscious processes to understand current behaviors and feelings. Reflecting on past emotional memories and the conceptual frameworks around them aligns with the introspective nature of this therapy.
Step 3 Committing to consciousness	1. Daily Intentional Consciousness	1/2. MBSR and MBCT Why: The daily intention setting and regular check-ins are ways of cultivating mindfulness in day-to-day life, allowing individuals to be more present and aware.
Step 4 An unconscious inventory	1. Conscious Values Assessment 2. Generational Unconscious Analysis 3. Soma Assessment 4. Sentence Completion 5. Concept Evolution Evaluation	1. Acceptance and Commitment Therapy (ACT) Why: ACT involves clarifying one's values and taking action that is consistent with these values. By reflecting on personal values and how they guide behavior, individuals are practicing an essential component of ACT. 2. Psychoanalytic/Psychodynamic Therapy Why: This modality delves deep into early experiences, often within the family of origin, to understand how past dynamics influence present behavior. By exploring generational beliefs and behaviors, individuals tap into insights about the unconscious patterns and defense mechanisms that might have been passed down or developed in response to family dynamics.

		3. Somatic Experiencing (SE)
		Why: This is a therapeutic approach developed by Dr. Peter Levine that emphasizes bodily sensations to heal trauma. Recognizing and sitting with bodily sensations, as suggested in the exercise, aligns with this modality's principles of healing through bodily awareness.
		4. Cognitive Behavioral Therapy (CBT)
		Why: Automatic thoughts and beliefs are central concepts in CBT. The sentence completion exercise helps surface these automatic thoughts, and challenging them aligns with CBT's approach to modifying dysfunctional thoughts.
		5. Schema Therapy
		Why: This modality emphasizes identifying and challenging deeply held beliefs (or schemas) that drive behaviors. Evaluating personal concepts and schemas aligns with the introspective and challenging nature of Schema Therapy.
Step 5 Conscious honesty	1. Conscious Self-Admission (Meditative/Mindful) 2. Unconscious Inventory Share	1. DBT Why: Mindfulness is one of the core components of DBT. The introspective exercises in Step 5 resonate with DBT's emphasis on observing and describing emotions and experiences without judgment.
		2. Group Therapy/Support Groups
		Why: The dynamic of sharing personal experiences in a group setting, where members provide feedback and insights, or simply listen, mirrors the process of the Unconscious Inventory Share. It emphasizes the therapeutic power of sharing and receiving feedback in a supportive environment.

Step 6 Prep yourself	1. Unconscious Change List 2. Short List: Unconscious Changes	1. SE Why: These approaches focus on the connection between the mind and the body. Recognizing somatic patterns, such as neglecting physical health or bodily tension reactivity, aligns directly with the principles of this therapy. Metacognitive Therapy (MCT) Why: MCT is all about understanding one's thinking about thinking (or metacognition). Recognizing repetitive thought patterns or automatic negative self-talk is a step toward this awareness. Psychoanalytic/Psychodynamic Therapy Why: Recognizing behaviors like avoidance of self-reflection or repetition of unhealthy patterns echoes the core principles of this therapy.
Step 7 Conscious Control and Change	Conscious Growth Action Plan	Somatic Sensorimotor Psychotherapy Why: Sensorimotor Psychotherapy combines talk therapy with body-centered approaches. The focus on "interoceptive attunement" and "body movement/activation" aligns with this modality's emphasis on using the body (somatic experiences) to inform cognitive and emotional processing. Cognitive CBT Why: CBT focuses on the relationship between thoughts, feelings, and behaviors. The "intention setting" and "first thought, second thought (metacognition)" components of Step 7 echo CBT's approach of identifying and reframing maladaptive thought patterns to produce positive behavioral change.

		Psychoanalytic
		Psychodynamic Therapy
		Why: Psychodynamic therapy explores unconscious processes as they manifest in a person's present behavior. The "supportive statements" and "storytelling" components reflect the modality's emphasis on understanding and interpreting past experiences, internal conflicts, and the unconscious mind.
		Environment/Supports
		No direct Evidence-Based Practice (EBP), general recommendations.
Step 8 Unconscious harms	1. Unconscious Amends List	1. No direct EBP, general 12-Step recommendation
Step 9 Acts of amends	1. Acts of Amends	1. DBT Why: DBT is a form of CBT that focuses on developing skills for emotional regulation, interpersonal effectiveness, distress tolerance, and mindfulness. The Step 9 experience emphasizes emotional introspection, active listening, and effective interpersonal communication—particularly in making direct amends. Furthermore, the emphasis on self-reflection and affirmations in the experience aligns with the mindfulness and emotional regulation components of DBT.
Step 10 Ongoing self-consciousness	1. Conscious Human Self-Assessment	1. MBCT Why: MBCT combines traditional cognitive behavioral approaches with mindfulness strategies. It aims to break the link between automatic and reactive thinking patterns, particularly for individuals with recurring depression.

		Many questions in Step 10 revolve around self-awareness and under-standing one's thinking patterns, such as "What judgments and biases did you engage in?" The core of mindfulness is about being present and aware without judgment, which aligns with the intro-spection encouraged in this step.
Step 11 Further your conscious un-derstanding	1. Metta Meditation 2. Yoga or Another Body-Based Move-ment 3. Continuous Learn-ing and Exploration 4. Community and/or Spiritual Engagement 5. Conscious Cultural Expansion	1. MBSR/MBCT Why: Both MBSR and MBCT centralize mindfulness meditation to cultivate a heightened awareness of present thoughts and feelings. The meditation and breath awareness advocated in Step 11's "meditation and mindfulness" echo the foundational principles of MBSR and MBCT, focusing on nonjudg-mental observation and presence. 2. Body Psychotherapy Why: Body Psychotherapy emphasizes the intrinsic connection between the physical body, emotions, and cognition. Step 11's "yoga or another body-based movement" encourages alignment of breath and movement and a deeper understanding of physical sensations, mirroring the holistic approach of Body Psychotherapy. 3/4/5. No direct EBP, general con-sciousness growth recommendations.
Step 12 Shared con-sciousness	1. Conscious Support	1. No direct EBP, general 12-Step recommendation.

Glossary of Terms

I have organized these terms alphabetically. The definitions used are specific to the context and intention of the book's messaging.

Acceptance and Commitment Therapy (ACT): A therapeutic approach helping individuals embrace their thoughts and feelings rather than fighting or feeling guilty for them.

Allostasis: Your body's ability to achieve stability and physiologically adapt through change, particularly in response to stress.

Amygdala: A part of the brain involved in processing emotions and determining potential threats.

Archetypes: Universal symbols or patterns that are part of the collective unconscious, as proposed by Jung.

Behavioral Mimicry: When you unconsciously imitate or copy the behaviors of others.

Borderline Personality Disorder (BPD): A mental health condition characterized by unstable moods, self-image, and interpersonal relationships, often leading to impulsive actions and intense emotional reactions.

Cognitive Interpretation: How your brain understands and labels your bodily sensations.

Cognitive Miser: A term that describes your brain's tendency to seek short-cuts in decision-making.

Cognitive Unconscious: The mental perceptions and information processing that occur within your brain without your conscious awareness or control.

Collective Unconscious: Jung's theory that we have memories and ideas inherited from our ancestors, common to all humans.

Concepts: Mental constructs that help you categorize, understand, and simplify the vast information your mind takes in.

Conscious Emotions: Emotions you are acutely aware of. See *Feelings*.

Conscious, Preconscious, Unconscious Mind: Freud's model of the mind, where the conscious is your immediate awareness, the preconscious holds retrievable memories not currently in focus, and the unconscious stores your repressed memories and feelings beyond easy access.

Consciously Curated Unconscious: A three-part unconscious that is actively understood, intentionally molded, and held consciously responsible.

Consciousness: Awareness of your own existence, sensations, and environment; the feeling and knowing of what happens.

Counterfactuals: When you think about alternative scenarios to past events in your life.

Courage: The willingness to confront and embrace your unconscious parts, even when it challenges your comfort zones or beliefs.

Death: The permanent stopping of all critical life functions.

Defense Mechanisms: Freud's concept that our minds employ certain strategies to avoid confronting distressing unconscious thoughts.

Dissociation: A physiological and psychological experience in which people disconnect from their sensory experience, sense of self, or personal history.

Dopamine: A neurotransmitter responsible for pleasure, motivation, and reward sensations.

Downward Counterfactuals: When you imagine how a situation could have been worse.

Drunkard's Search Principle: The idea that people tend to look for answers where it's easiest rather than where the answers might actually be found.

Emotion: The interplay between our body's raw physiological reactions and our brain's conscious or unconscious interpretation of these sensations in context.

Emotional Contagion: The unconscious transfer of emotions between you and other people.

Explicit Memory: Conscious recall of facts, events, or knowledge.

Fear Conditioning: A form of learning where a neutral stimulus becomes associated with a fear response after being paired with an aversive stimulus.

Feelings: Your conscious experience of emotional states; what you are actively aware of and can articulate.

Fundamental Human Motives: Deeply ingrained drivers that influence your behavior based on evolutionary needs.

Generational Trauma: The transmission of historical and collective trauma from one generation to another, often impacting individuals' mental, emotional, and social well-being.

Generational Unconscious: The transfer of historical and collective unconscious behaviors, emotions, feelings, and judgments from one generation to another.

Homeostasis: Your body's natural tendency to maintain stability or equilibrium in its internal environment.

Human Paradox: The more you admit being a human is hard, the easier it becomes to be one.

Id, Ego, Superego: Freud's model of personality, where the id represents primitive desires, the ego is the conscious self, and the superego is our internal moral compass.

Implicit Memory: Memories that operate below your conscious awareness, influencing your behavior.

Individuation: Jung's process of becoming the person one inherently is, by integrating different parts of one's personality.

Interoception: The perception and awareness of your body's sensations and signals.

Law of Control: The principle suggesting that your emotional well-being is linked to your perceived control over life events.

Learned Helplessness: A theory suggesting that after repeated negative experiences that are out of one's control, an individual learns to behave helplessly, not even trying to avoid the negative situation when it becomes avoidable.

Locus of Control: A psychological concept that determines whether you feel in control of your own fate (internal), if external factors are in control (external), or the control is shared (mixed).

Long-Term Memory: Memory storage that can last from days to a lifetime.

Mechanoreception: Your body's ability to detect touch and pressure.

Memories: Snapshots of past emotional states captured in both body and brain, shaping your behaviors and decisions.

Metta: A state of positive energy and kindness toward oneself and others.

Mind: The part of you containing your feelings, thoughts, and consciousness.

Misattribution of Arousal: Mistaking bodily arousal for a particular feeling, like thinking fear is romantic attraction.

Near-Death Experience: A profound psychological event that may occur to someone close to death or in extreme physical or emotional crisis.

Neuroadaptation: When your brain adjusts to the presence of a stimulus, often leading to tolerance or dependence on substances or other types of behaviors.

Nociception: The somatic sensory process that provides the signals that lead to your perception of pain.

Nonverbal Communication: How you convey information without words, for example through body language.

Objective Helplessness: A situation where actions genuinely do not change the outcome, making you behaviorally and probabilistically powerless.

OxyContin: A potent opioid painkiller introduced by Purdue Pharma in 1995.

Pain–Pleasure Principle: An inherent human trait where actions are driven by the pursuit of pleasure and avoidance of pain.

Physiological Arousal: Physical reactions like increased heart rate or sweating.

Post-Traumatic Stress Disorder (PTSD): A mental health condition triggered by experiencing or witnessing a traumatic event, characterized by recurrent, distressing memories, avoidance behaviors, and heightened arousal reactions.

Priming: A cognitive process where exposure to a stimulus unconsciously influences a response to a subsequent stimulus.

Proprioception: Your body's ability to sense its position in space.

Prototypes: Standard or typical examples that best represent a category or a concept.

Psychoanalysis: A form of therapy that attempts to access someone's unconscious mind or "subconscious" in order to treat mental health conditions.

Psychoanalytic Unconscious: The experiential outcomes that influence you without your conscious awareness or control.

Psychoanalyze: To examine someone's mind to understand their thoughts and behaviors.

Reverse Inference Problem: The difficulty of deducing specific mental states from brain activity.

Serenity: A state of calm acceptance and understanding of your unconscious, allowing for clearer self-awareness and mental peace.

Shadow: In Jung's theory, it refers to the parts of our personality we don't recognize or appreciate. It is the source of our biases and prejudices.

Short-Term Memory (Working Memory): Temporary memory storage for your current tasks or processes.

Situational and Contextual Features: Elements or factors that define a particular situation or context that unconsciously influence your behaviors and decisions.

Somatic Experiencing: A therapy focusing on bodily sensations to heal trauma.

Somatic Sensory Integration: The process by which your brain receives, interprets, and responds to the messages sent by the somatic unconscious.

Somatic Unconscious: The bodily reactions and sensations that occur within your body and brain without your conscious awareness or control.

Subjective Helplessness: The cognitive recognition and internalization of the belief that your actions cannot alter negative outcomes in your life.

Thermoception: Your body's ability to sense warmth or coldness.

Third-Person Mirror: An exercise in which you record your actions and interactions for a period of time, then review the footage to observe your nonverbal behaviors.

Thoughts: The ideas, images, beliefs, and opinions in your mind.

Turn On, Tune In, Drop Out, and Be Here Now: Timothy Leary's and Ram Dass's famously coined phrases combined to create reminders for the 12 Steps of Consciousness journey.

Two-Factor Theory of Emotion: Developed by Schachter and Singer (1960s); the idea that emotions come from a mix of bodily sensations and our understanding of them.

The Unconscious: The parts of you that function without your conscious awareness or control.

Unconscious Emotion: Emotions experienced without conscious awareness, influencing your thoughts and behaviors automatically.

Unconscious Paradox: The more you accept you're unconscious, the less unconscious you become.

Upward Counterfactuals: When you imagine how a situation could have turned out better.

Vegetative State: A state in which a person appears to be awake and their eyes may even be open, but they lack any form of conscious awareness; "wakefulness without awareness."

Wisdom: The ability to discern and navigate between your unconscious and consciousness, guiding healthier emotional and behavioral outcomes.

Notes

1: The New Three-Part Unconscious

1. Hopefully, this statement implies that, as therapists, we understand that we do not, cannot, and should not control our clients. Why? Because forces beyond our control (and our clients' control) impact their decisions, behaviors, thoughts, and feelings. Therapy is about people learning how to control themselves.

2. U.S. Department of Health and Human Services. (n.d.). *Borderline Personality Disorder*. National Institute of Mental Health, https://www.nimh.nih.gov/health/topics /borderline-personality-disorder.

3. E. Morsella, C. A. Godwin, T. K. Jantz, S. C. Krieger, and A. Gazzaley, "Homing In on Consciousness in the Nervous System: An Action-based Synthesis," *Behavioral and Brain Sciences* 39 (2016): https://doi.org/10.1017/S0140525X15000643.

4. J. Kluger, "Why You're Pretty Much Unconscious All the Time," *TIME*, June 26, 2015.

5. Julian B. Rotter, "Generalized Expectancies for Internal Versus External Control of Reinforcement," *Psychological Monographs: General and Applied* 80, no. 1 (1966): 1–28.

6. The four questions listed here have been adapted and developed from Patricia Dutt-weiler. The Internal Locus of Control Index (ICI) (1984) by Patricia Duttweiler is a twenty-eight-item instrument designed to measure where a person looks for, or expects to obtain, reinforcement; P. C. Duttweiler, "The Internal Control Index: A Newly Developed Measure of Locus of Control." *Educational and Psychological Measurement* 44, no. 2 (1984): 209–221.

7. The Alcoholics Anonymous (AA) adaptation of the serenity prayer was revised from the original; it was first written for sermons in the 1930s by Reinhold Niebuhr, an American theologian. It began to be used in the rooms of AA in the 1940s.

8. In this study, it was shown that the desire for a mate can sometimes supercede one's awareness of health risks associated with attractiveness-enhancing behaviors: S. E.

Hill and K. M. Durante, "Courtship, Competition, and the Pursuit of Attractiveness: Mating Goals Facilitate Health-Related Risk Taking and Strategic Risk Suppression in Women," *Personality and Social Psychology Bulletin* 37, no. 3 (2011): 383–394.

9.   D. C. Branson, "Vicarious Trauma, Themes in Research, and Terminology: A Review of Literature," *Traumatology* 25, no. 1 (2019): 2–10.

10.   F. Azevedo, S. Middleton, J. M. Phan, S. Kapp, A. Gourdon-Kanhukamwe, B. Iley, M. Elsherif, and J. J. Shaw, "Navigating Academia as Neurodivergent Researchers: Promoting Neurodiversity Within Open Scholarship," *Observer*, October 31, 2022, https://www.psychologicalscience.org/observer/gs-navigating-academia-as -neurodivergent-researchers.

2: You're Thinking About It All Wrong

1.   This metaphor was first used by Anita Moorjani in her book *Dying to Be Me* and her TED Talk with the same title. While doctors and Anita's family thought she had fallen into a state of comatose after a terminal cancer diagnosis and rapidly declining health, she was actually experiencing a super-state of heightened consciousness—one she would live to tell about; A. Moorjani, *Dying to Be Me: My Journey from Cancer, to Near Death, to True Healing* (Carlsbad, CA: Hay House, 2012).

2.   This telling of the warehouse metaphor is a combined and condensed version of both Anita's book and TED Talk versions.

3.   Many people who attempt the quick route through non-therapeutically adminstered drugs, the non–near-death experience "floodlight" route, end up traumatized from the lack of control they experience during their hours-long psychedelic trip. At the same time, there can be beautiful and very healing experiences that take place using these substances, which 100 percent require medical clearance of some kind, a proper environment, supervision, guidance, safety guidelines, and more.

4.   This is a very stereotypical description of a "hippie," although I'd argue that, technically, "hippie," in itself, is an overall stereotype at this point and not an actual type of person. Regardless, it should be noted that this description was intentionally exaggerated to make my point.

5.   J. Bargh, "How Unconscious Thought and Perception Affect Our Every Waking Moment," *Scientific American*, January 1, 2014.

6.   Bargh, "How Unconscious Thought and Perception."

7.   S. Schneider and M. Velmans, M. eds., *The Blackwell Companion to Consciousness*, 2nd ed. (Hoboken, NJ: Wiley-Blackwell, 2017).

8.   While this isn't the *most* academic source, I believe this is a helpful resource for the typical reader wanting to learn more about this deeply complex concept: IEP, "The Hard Problem of Consciousness," *Internet Encyclopedia of Philosophy* (n.d.), accessed August 9, 2024, https://iep.utm.edu/hard-problem-of-conciousness/.

9.   Gary D. Ellis, Judith E. Voelkl, and Catherine Morris, "Measurement and Analysis Issues with Explanation of Variance in Daily Experience Using the Flow Model," *Journal of Leisure Research* 26, no. 4 (1994): 337–356.

10.   John Green (@johngreenwritesbooks), Threads, July 21, 2023, https://www.threads .net/@johngreenwritesbooks.

11.   Antonio Damasio, *Feeling and Knowing: Making Minds Conscious* (New York, NY: Vintage Books, 2022).

12.   The Buddhist text *Tittha Sutta, Udāna 6.4, Khuddaka Nikaya* contains one of the

earliest versions of the story. The *Tittha Sutta* is dated to around 500 BCE. I adjusted this parable to fit the style of my writing. I highly encourage a review of some of the original tellings.

13. René Descartes (1596–1650): Descartes is known for his famous dictum "Cogito, ergo sum" (I think, therefore I am). He emphasized the certainty of self-awareness as the foundation of knowledge. Descartes's dualism posited a distinction between mind (res cogitans) and body (res extensa), suggesting that consciousness and physical reality were separate substances.

14. John Locke (1632–1704): Locke's "An Essay Concerning Human Understanding" (1689) is a foundational work in empiricism. He argued that all knowledge is derived from sensory experience and that consciousness is a tabula rasa—a blank slate—upon which experience writes.

15. Friedrich Nietzsche (1844–1900): Nietzsche's work delved into the complexities of consciousness, morality, and the human condition. He critiqued traditional philosophical approaches and explored the nature of individual perception and interpretation.

16. Michael Craig Miller, "Unconscious or Subconscious?," *Harvard Health Blog*, Harvard Health Publishing, August 2, 2010, https://www.health.harvard.edu/blog/unconscious-or-subconscious-20100801255.

17. Maxwell Kuzma (@maxwellkuzma), comment on John Green's post, Threads, July 24, 2023, https://www.threads.net/@maxwellkuzma/post/CvF3r1aPgqC.

18. M. Velmans, "Conscious Agency and the Preconscious/Unconscious Self," in *Interdisciplinary Perspectives on Consciousness and the Self*, eds. Sangeetha Menon, Anindya Sinha, B. V. Sreekantan (New Delhi: Springer, 2014), 11–25.

19. D. K. Lapsley, and P. C. Stey, (n.d.). "Id, Ego, and Superego," https://www3.nd.edu/~dlapsle1/Lab/Articles_&_Chapters_files/Entry%20for%20Encyclopedia%20of%20Human%20BehaviorFInal%20Submitted%20Formatted4.pdf.

20. Marie Kuhfuß, Tobias Maldei, Andreas Hetmanek, and Nicola Baumann, "Somatic Experiencing—Effectiveness and Key Factors of a Body-Oriented Trauma Therapy: A Scoping Literature Review," *European Journal of Psychotraumatology* 12, no. 1 (2021): 1929023.

21. J. Fisher, "Sensorimotor Psychotherapy in the Treatment of Trauma," *Practice Innovations* 4, no. 3 (2019): 156–165.

22. M. McKee, "Biofeedback: An Overview in the Context of Heart-Brain Medicine," *Cleveland Clinic Journal of Medicine* 75, no. 2 (2008): S31–S34.

23. Paul Rozin is credited with having coined the term "cognitive unconscious." Super thankful for this contribution. P. Rozin, "The Evolution of Intelligence and Access to the Cognitive Unconscious," *Progress of Psychobiology and Physiological Psychology* 6 (1976): 245–280.

24. T. Soondrum, X. Wang, F. Gao, Q. Liu, J. Fan, and X. Zhu, "The Applicability of Acceptance and Commitment Therapy for Obsessive-Compulsive Disorder: A Systematic Review and Meta-analysis," *Brain Sciences* 12, no. 5 (2022): 656.

25. K. Bilodeau, "Managing Intrusive Thoughts," *Mind & Mood*, Harvard Health Publishing, March 26, 2024, https://www.health.harvard.edu/mind-and-mood/managing-intrusive-thoughts.

26. J. Shedler, "That Was Then, This Is Now: Psychoanalytic Psychotherapy for the Rest of Us," *Contemporary Psychoanalysis* 58, no. 2–3 (2022): 405–437.

27. Center for Substance Abuse Treatment, "Chapter 7—Brief Psychodynamic Therapy,"

in *Treatment Improvement Protocols* (Rockville, MD: Substance Abuse and Mental Health Services Administration, 1999).

28. H. S. Baker and M. N. Baker, "Heinz Kohut's Self Psychology: An Overview," *American Journal of Psychiatry* 144, no. 1 (1987): 1–9.

29. A. Gopnik, "Why Babies Are More Conscious than We Are," *Behavioral and Brain Sciences* 30, no. 5–6 (2007): 503–504.

30. C. Trevarthen and V. Reddy, "Consciousness in Infants," in *The Blackwell Companion to Consciousness*, eds. Susan Schneider and Max Velmans (Hoboken, NJ: John Wiley & Sons, 2017): 43–62.

31. Claire Hannah Collins and Ada Tseng, "How My Mental Illness Became My Superpower," *The Los Angeles Times*, October 5, 2021. I'd like to note here that I stand by any person using any (non-subjectively/objectively-harmful) language and conceptualization to heal and progress in their own mental health recovery. I'm so glad it's been helpful.

32. Wikipedia, "Jazz Thornton," last modified February 5, 2024, https://en.wikipedia.org/wiki/Jazz_Thornton.

3: What You Feel Is What You Think

1. This was three years post Chapter One's diagnosis and ultimatum.

2. Barring any sinus differences or other sensory ailments.

3. T. Hanna, "What Is Somatics?," *Somatics: Magazine-Journal of the Bodily Arts and Sciences* 5, no. 4 (1986): 4–8.

4. N. Fattorini, C. Brunetti, C. Baruzzi, E, Macchi, M. C. Pagliarella, N. Pallari, S. Lovari, and F. Ferretti, "Being 'Hangry': Food Depletion and Its Cascading Effects on Social Behaviour," *Biological Journal of the Linnean Society* 125, no. 3 (2018): 640–656.

5. A. V. Apkarian, "Definitions of Nociception, Pain, and Chronic Pain with Implications Regarding Science and Society," *Neuroscience Letters* 702 (2019): 1–2.

6. A. Vabba, M. S. Panasiti, M. Scattolin, M. Spitaleri, G. Porciello, and S. M. Aglioti, "The Thermoception Task: A Thermal-Imaging Based Procedure for Measuring Awareness of Changes in Peripheral Body Temperature," *Journal of Neurophysiology* 130, no. 4 (2023): 1053–1064.

7. J. Munóz-Jiménez, D. Rojas-Valverde, and K. Leon, "Future Challenges in the Assessment of Proprioception in Exercise Sciences: Is Imitation an Alternative?," *Frontiers in Human Neuroscience* 15 (2021): 644667.

8. A. Prochazka, "Proprioception: Clinical Relevance and Neurophysiology," *Current Opinion in Physiology* 23 (2021): 100440.

9. B. E. Kearney and R. A. Lanius, "The Brain-Body Disconnect: A Somatic Sensory Basis for Trauma-Related Disorders," *Frontiers in Neuroscience* 16 (2022):1015749.

10. Abby Hershler, Lesley Hughes, Patricia Nguyen, and Shelley Wall, eds., *Looking at Trauma: A Tool Kit for Clinicians* (University Park: Penn State University Press, 2021). This is a great tool kit in which the Window of Tolerance is explicitly addressed in Chapter 4.

11. B. S. McEwen, "The Untapped Power of Allostasis Promoted by Healthy Lifestyles," *World Psychiatry: Official Journal of the World Psychiatric Association (WPA)* 19, no. 1 (2020): 57–58.

12. W. G. Chen, D. Schloesser, A. M. Arensdorf, J. M. Simmons, C. Cui, R. Valentino,

J. W. Gnadt, L. Nielsen, C. St Hillaire-Clarke, V. Spruaance, T. S. Horowitz, Y. F. Vallejo, and H. M. Langevin, "The Emerging Science of Interoception: Sensing, Integrating, Interpreting, and Regulating Signals within the Self," *Trends in Neurosciences* 44, no. 1 (2021): 3–16.

13. K. Armstrong, " Interoception: How We Understand Our Body's Inner Sensations," *Observer,* September 25, 2019, https://www.psychologicalscience.org/observer/interoception-how-we-understand-our-bodys-inner-sensations.

14. J. A. Hall, T. G. Horgan, and N. A. Murphy, "Nonverbal Communication," *Annual Review of Psychology* 70, no. 1 (2019): 271–294.

15. It should be noted that Emily confirmed these somatic behaviors were, in fact, unconscious. She did not consciously decide to roll her eyes, take off her jacket, or adjust her seat. She just did them. These are all behaviors that can be consciously controlled, yes, but in many cases, they aren't. Like this one.

16. Spidey-sense is a precognitive ability that allows Spider-Man to sense danger before it happens. It is a powerful ability that has saved Spider-Man's life countless times. It doesn't apply specifically, but it worked well enough.

17. D. G. Dutton and A. P. Aaron, "Some Evidence for Heightened Sexual Attraction under Conditions of High Anxiety," *Journal of Personality and Social Psychology* 30, no. 4 (1974): 510–517.

18. O. E. Dror, "Deconstructing the 'Two Factors': The Historical Origins of the Schachter–Singer Theory of Emotions," *Emotion Review: Journal of the International Society for Research on Emotion* 9, no. 1 (2017): 7–16.

4: You Are Biased

1. J. Stromberg, "The Neuroscientist Who Discovered He Was a Psychopath," *Smithsonian,* November 22, 2013.

2. W. J. Shoemaker, *The Origin of Evil and the Social Brain Network* (Meadville, PA: Fulton Books, 2023).

3. A. J. R. Galang, "The Prosocial Psychopath: Explaining the Paradoxes of the Creative Personality," *Neuroscience and Biobehavioral Reviews* 34, no. 8 (2010): 1241–1248.

4. A. I. Jack, K. C. Rochford, J. P. Friedman, A. M. Passarelli, and R. E. Boyatzis, "Pitfalls in Organizational Neuroscience: A Critical Review and Suggestions for Future Research," *Organizational Research Methods* 22, no. 1 (2019): 421–458.

5. Stromberg, "The Neuroscientist Who Discovered He Was a Psychopath."

6. C. E. L. Stark, "Truth, Lies, and False Memories: Neuroscience in the Courtroom," *Dana Foundation: Report on Progress,* 2014.

7. A. Kaplan, *The Conduct of Inquiry: Methodology for Behavioral Science* (New Brunswick, NJ: Transaction Publishers, 1964).

8. David H. Freedman, *Wrong: Why Experts Keep Failing Us* (New York, NY: Little, Brown and Company, 2010).

9. S. Frederick, "Cognitive Reflection and Decision Making," *Journal of Economic Perspectives* 19 (2005): 25–42. This is one of the most common experiential examples used to showcase human cognition.

10. U. Bockenholt, "The Cognitive-Miser Response Model: Testing for Intuitive and Deliberate Reasoning," *Psychometrika* 77 (2012): 388–399.

11. Juli Weiner, "Fuck, Marry, Kill: 'First Daughter, First Love' Edition!" *Wonkette,* April 14, 2009.

12. S. M. Kassin, S. Fein, and H. R. Markus, *Social Psychology,* 8th ed. (Belmont, CA: Wadsworth Publishing, 2010).

13. Cognitive miserliness was first proposed as a model for human thinking in 1984 by psychologists Susan Fiske and Shelley Taylor in their book *Social Cognition.*

14. K. J. Holyoak and R. G. Morrison, *The Oxford Handbook of Thinking and Reasoning* (Oxford: Oxford University Press, 2013).

15. J. Fukuta and J. Yamashita, "The Complex Relationship between Conscious/Unconscious Learning and Conscious/Unconscious Knowledge: The Mediating Effects of Salience in Form–Meaning Connections," *Second Language Research* 39, no. 2 (2023): 425–446.

16. Richard Crisp and Rhiannon Turner, *Essential Social Psychology,* 4th ed. (Thousand Oaks, CA: Sage Publications, 2020).

17. S.-M. Lee, R. N. Henson, and C.-Y. Lin, "Neural Correlates of Repetition Priming: A Coordinate-Based Meta-Analysis of fMRI Studies," *Frontiers in Human Neuroscience* 14 (2020): 565114.

18. L. Grégoire, I. Gosselin, and I. Blanchette, "The Impact of Trauma Exposure on Explicit and Implicit Memory," *Anxiety, Stress, and Coping* 33, no. 1 (2020): 1–18.

19. I. Rehman, N. Mahabadi, T., Sanvictores, and C. I. Rehman, *Classical Conditioning* (Tampa, FL: StatPearls Publishing, 2023).

20. Stephen R. Tarbell, "Democratic Voters Are Sheep," Letters, *Boston Globe,* September 18, 2014.

21. K. M. Junior, "The Sheer Hypocrisy of Republicans Referring to Democrats as Sheep," *Medium,* July 9, 2022.

22. "Which Party, Democrat or Republican, Has the Most Sheep?" Quora (n.d.).

23. Definition of *sheeple.* Merriam-webster.com (n.d.).

24. A. Pereira, "Merriam-Webster Defines 'Sheeple' Using Apple Fans as Example," *San Francisco Chronicle,* May 1, 2017.

25. This is a lot of shit-talking on iPhone users. I've wastefully had over twenty iPhones in my life. I love Apple products. I am an Apple sheep. I'm working on it.

26. M. Zetlin, "Love Apple products? Merriam-Webster Says You're a 'Sheeple,'" *Inc.,* April 29, 2017.

27. It should be noted that the phenomenon of suicide contagion does not indicate a need to reduce the public awareness and open conversations about suicide that have been increasing in our country. Talking to people about their suicidal ideation or behaviors has not been shown to cause individuals to feel more suicidal.

28. C. B. Zhong and K. Lijenquist, "Washing Away Your Sins: Threatened Mortality and Physical Cleansing," *Science* 313 (2006): 1451–1452.

29. H. Aarts and A. Dijksterhuis, "The Silence of the Library: Environment, Situational Norm, and Social Behavior," *Journal of Personality and Social Psychology* 84, no.1 (2003): 18–28.

30. R. W. Holland, M. Hendriks, and H. Aarts, "Smells like Clean Spirit: Nonconscious Effects of Scent on Cognition and Behavior," *Psychological Science* 16, no. 9 (2005): 689–693.

31. C. Jacob, N. Guéguen, A. Martin, and G. Boulbry, "Retail Salespeople's Mimicry of Customers: Effects on Consumer Behavior," *Journal of Retailing and Consumer Services* 18, no. 5 (2011): 381–388.

32. V. Griskevicius, and D. T. Kenrick, "Fundamental Motives: How Evolutionary Needs Influence Consumer Behavior," *Journal of Consumer Psychology: The Official Journal of the Society for Consumer Psychology* 23, no. 3 (2013): 372–386.

33. S. Schnall, J. Haiti, J., G. L. Clore, and A. H. Jordan, "Disgust as Embodied Moral Judgment," *Personality and Social Psychology Bulletin* 34 (2008): 1096–1109.

34. Schnall, et al.

35. In this study, it was shown that the desire for a mate can sometimes supercede one's awareness of health risks associated with attractiveness-enhancing behaviors: S. E. Hill and K. M. Durante, "Courtship, Competition, and the Pursuit of Attractiveness: Mating Goals Facilitate Health-Related Risk Taking and Strategic Risk Suppression in Women," *Personality and Social Psychology Bulletin* 37, no. 3 (2011): 383–394.

36. J. Hermans, H. Slabbinck, J. Vanderstraeten, J. Brassey, M. Dejardin, D. Ramdani, and A. Van Witteloostuijin, "The Power Paradox: Implicit and Explicit Power Motives, and the Importance Attached to Prosocial Organizational Goals in SMEs," *Sustainability* 9 (2017): 1–26.

37. M. Lenzen, "Feeling Our Emotions," *Scientific American Mind* 16, no. 1 (2005): 14–15.

38. Lenzen, "Feeling Our Emotions."

5: Who You Are Is a Concept

1. In vitro fertilization, or IVF, is a way to help couples have a baby when they are unable to do so naturally.

2. To be honest, I don't remember the details, but I'm sure the argument was something about communication and fairness as we were struggling with them at the time.

3. Some would say this could have been a "trauma reenactment," where Max may have been unconsciously 0—repeating experiences similar to original traumas he'd been through.

4. Delusions can be complex and can vary in their presentation and impact.

5. D. DiSalvo, "Your Brain Sees Even When You Don't," *Forbes*, June 22, 2013.

6. K. I. Al-Malah, "The Human Brain: Search for Natural Intelligence," *International Journal of Educational Policy Research and Review* 8, no. 6 (2021): 232–235.

7. J. E. LeDoux, "Emotion and the Amygdala," in *The Amygdala: Neurobiological Aspects of Emotion, Memory, and Mental Dysfunction*, J. P. Aggleton, ed. (New York, NY: Wiley-Liss, 1992), 339–351.

8. I never said I didn't like Freud or his theories (although some are absolutely ridiculous). I said I didn't like the word "subconscious" because of how it limited the general population's thinking around what controls us outside of our awareness. Freud was a great thinker of his time using the tools he had, along with the limited mental and physical health he was clearly dealing with.

9. A. L. Baxter, A. Thrasher, J. L. Etnoyer-Slaski, and L. L. Cohen, "Multimodal Mechanical Stimulation Reduces Acute and Chronic Low Back Pain: Pilot Data from a HEAL Phase 1 Study," *Frontiers in Pain Research* 4 (2023): 1114633.

10. A. Lembke, *Dopamine Nation: Finding Balance in the Age of Indulgence* (New York, NY: Dutton, 2021).

11. J. C. Ballantyne and G. F. Koob, "Allostasis Theory in Opioid Tolerance," *Pain* 162, no. 9 (2021): 2315–2319.

12. N. Van Hoeck, P. D. Watson, and A. K. Barbey, "Cognitive Neuroscience of Human Counterfactual Reasoning," *Frontiers in Human Neuroscience* 9 (2015): 420.

13. Van Hoeck, Watson, and Barbey, "Cognitive Neuroscience of Human Counterfactual Reasoning."

14. It's worth noting that while these patterns of counterfactual thinking are common,

individual and cultural differences may influence how people engage in this type of thinking.

15.   V. Husted Medvec, S. F. Madey, and T. Gilovich, "When Less Is More: Counterfactual Thinking and Satisfaction among Olympic Medalists," in *Social Cognition* (New York, NY: Psychology Press, 2004), 579–588.

16.   N. J. Roese, and J. M. Olson, eds., *What Might Have Been: The Social Psychology of Counterfactual Thinking* (New York, NY: Psychology Press, 1995).

17.   L. J. Sanna, K. J. Turley-Ames, and S. Meier, "Mood, Self-esteem, and Simulated Alternatives: Thought-Provoking Affective Influences on Counterfactual Direction," *Journal of Personality and Social Psychology* 76, no. 4 (1999): 543–558.

18.   R. M. J. Byrne, "Counterfactual Thought," *Annual Review of Psychology* 67, no. 1 (2016): 135–157.

19.   The majority of this section has been sourced from the following article written by Maier and Seligman themselves about realizing they had their own theory backward. It's worth the read: S. F. Maier, and M. E. P. Seligman, "Learned Helplessness at Fifty: Insights from Neuroscience," *Psychological Review* 123, no. 4 (2016): 349–367; It should be noted that my book is to be edgy and pushy. By this I mean no disrespect to these two individuals. Thank you both for your work, truly. I've been following your work for almost two decades.

20.   D. S. Hiroto, and M. E. Seligman, "Generality of Learned Helplessness in Man," *Journal of Personality and Social Psychology* 31, no. 2 (1975): 311–327.

6: Be a Human First

1.   Timothy Leary papers, New York Public Library, https://archives.nypl.org/mss/18400.

2.   Timothy Leary. (n.d.). "Timothy Leary: The Effects of Psychotropic Drugs," https://psychology.fas.harvard.edu/people/timothy-leary.

3.   *Turn On, Tune In, Drop Out*, directed by Robin S. Clark (1967).

4.   E. J. Fehr, and G. L. Sandelier, "Remember Be Here Now," in *Therapy*, S. S. Fehr, ed. (New York, NY: Routledge, 2010), 453–457.

5.   Both Timothy and Ram Dass followed their individual paths until the end of their days. Timothy, who faced legal battles and periods of incarceration due to his advocacy for psychedelics, passed away from inoperable cancer in 1996. Despite the controversies, his legacy continues to influence those who dare to challenge societal norms and explore the uncharted territories of consciousness. Ram Dass continued sharing his wisdom through his writing and teaching after a stroke in 1997. He embraced a life of service and passed away peacefully at home in 2019. His message of love, compassion, and mindfulness resonates with seekers of spiritual truth to this day.

6.   These first three were adapted from Timothy Leary's own account of what "Turn on, tune in, drop out" means from his 1983 autobiography *Flashbacks*.

7.   J. Bennett, "If Everything Is 'Trauma,' Is Anything?," *New York Times*, February 4, 2022.

8.   N. Haslam, and M. J. McGrath, "The Creeping Concept of Trauma," *Social Research* 87, no. 3 (2020): 509–531.

9.   Bessel van der Kolk, *The Body Keeps the Score: Brain, Mind, and Body in the Healing of Trauma* (New York: NY: Viking, 2014).

10.   First said differently by Brad Stulberg as "Fierce self-discipline requires fierce self-compassion."

7: See Yourself

1. Portia Nelson, *There's a Hole in My Sidewalk: The Romance of Self-Discovery* (New York, NY: Beyond Words Publishing, 1993).

2. A. W. Wu, "Medical Error: The Second Victim," *BMJ* 320, no. 7237 (2000): 726–727.

3. P. Phillips, *ASTD Handbook of Measuring and Evaluating Training* (Alexandria, VA: American Society for Training and Development, 2010).

4. C. Dweck, *Mindset: The New Psychology of Success* (New York, NY: Random House, 2017).

5. J. S. Moser, H. S. Schroder, C. Heeter, T. P. Moran, and Y.-H. Lee, "Mind Your Errors: Evidence for a Neural Mechanism Linking Growth Mind-set to Adaptive Post-error Adjustments," *Psychological Science* 22, no. 12 (2011): 1484–1489.

6. If you move forward with receiving the "human first" tattoo, please make sure you go to a reputable place and ensure they are licensed. Tattoos can be permanent (most are), and as much as you'll always be a human first, make sure you'll always want the tattoo before you get it.

8: Grow Consciously

1. I don't enjoy how much we've begun to use the word "toxic" in mental health and therapy language. Of course, yes, I have contributed to this pattern in many ways in the past—especially in my early online content. I hope we reduce the word's use moving forward, and replace the majority of its use with more nuanced words that directly explain the problematic nature of the behaviors being addressed.

2. Microagressions are subtle, often unintentional, actions or comments that can belittle or offend someone, usually related to their social or cultural identity. Examples: Asking a person of color, "Where are you really from?", implying they are not truly from their claimed country, or telling a woman, "You're pretty smart for a girl," suggesting women are typically not intelligent.

3. D. Schroeder and E. Gefenas, "Vulnerability: Too Vague and Too Broad?", *CQ: Cambridge Quarterly of Healthcare Ethics* 18, no. 2 (2009): 113–121.

9: Go In and Give Back

1. G. J. Annas, "'Culture of Life' Politics at the Bedside—The Case of Terri Schiavo," *New England Journal of Medicine* 352 (2005): 1710–1715.

2. B. Jennett and F. Plum, "Persistent Vegetative State after Brain Damage," *Lancet* 299, no. 7753 (1972): 734–737.

3. S. Laureys, "Death, Unconsciousness and the Brain," *Nature Reviews Neuroscience* 6, no. 11 (2005): 899–909.

4. J. Korein and C. Machado, "Brain Death," in *Brain Death and Disorders of Consciousness*, C. Machado and D. A. Shewmon, eds. (New York, NY: Kluwer Academic/Plenum, 2004).

5. S. Laureys, M.-E. Faymonville, X. De Tiège, P. Peigneux, J. Berré, G. Moonen, S. Goldman, and P. Maque, "Brain Function in the Vegetative State," *Advances in Experimental Medicine and Biology* 550 (2004): 229–238.

6. Over the past twelve years, I've come to understand the various forms of empathy. At the time of that statement, I was capable of what's called "cognitive empathy." I

understood human beings and how they could feel. However, I wasn't allowing *myself* to truly feel my own emotions, therefore I was limited in my ability to feel others' emotions, a phenomenon also known as "emotional empathy." I now have a full range of empathic abilities (to ease the mind of those of you concerned due to my profession).

7.   S. Stefan and S. G. Hofmann, "Integrating Metta into CBT: How Loving Kindness and Compassion Meditation Can Enhance CBT for Treating Anxiety and Depression," *Clinical Psychology in Europe* 1, no. 3 (2019): 1–15.

8.   A. Feliu-Soler, J. C. Pascual, M. Elices, A. Martín-Blanco, C. Carmona, A. Cebolla, V. Simón, and J. Soler, "Fostering Self-Compassion and Loving-Kindness in Patients with Borderline Personality Disorder: A Randomized Pilot Study," *Clinical Psychology and Psychotherapy* 24, no. 1 (2017): 278–286.

Index

About the Author

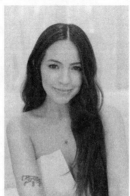

Truth Doctor Media

DR. COURTNEY TRACY, also known as The Truth Doctor, is a USC-trained psychotherapist recognized as one of the most authentic, perspective-shifting voices on mental health and the human condition and one of the first therapists to publicly disclose her own mental disorders. A multihyphenate healthcare entrepreneur and award-winning content creator, Tracy has founded five mental health companies and her work has garnered more than one hundred million views. She lives in Orange County, California.